CDT 2013

Dental Procedure Codes

ADA American Dental Association®
America's leading advocate for oral health

Table of Contents

Preface

Introduction

CDT 2013 is the reference manual published by the ADA that contains the *Code on Dental Procedures and Nomenclature* (CDT Code). This version of the CDT Code is effective for services provided on or after January 1, 2013 through December 31, 2013.

In August 2000 the CDT Code was designated by the federal government as the national terminology for reporting dental services on claims submitted to third-party payers, in accordance with authority granted by the Health Insurance Portability and Accountability Act of 1996 (HIPAA).

The ADA's Council on Dental Benefit Programs is responsible for maintaining the CDT Code in accordance with ADA Bylaws and policy, and applicable federal regulations. CDT Manual content is developed by the Council, while responsibility for CDT Manual printing, pricing and distribution of falls to the ADA's Department of Product Development and Sales.

- Should you have any recommendations for **additions, revisions or deletions** to the CDT Code, direct access to the process is available via the portal established on the ADA web page *ADA.org/3827.aspx.*

- **Technical questions** on the CDT Code or ADA Dental Claim Form should be directed to the ADA's Member Service Center (members: toll free number on your membership card; non-members: 312.440.2500).

- For general information about, or to pursue CDT Code **licensing,** please go to the ADA web page *ADA.org/3854.aspx.* In addition to information about licensing this site contains the questionnaire that must be completed as the first step of the licensing process.

- For any questions regarding **pricing or purchasing** additional copies of the CDT Manual visit *adacatalog.org* or call 800.947.4746.

Preface

Categories of Service

The CDT Code is organized into twelve categories of service, each with its own series of five-digit alphanumeric codes:

Category of Service		Code Series
I.	Diagnostic	D0100 – D0999
II.	Preventive	D1000 – D1999
III.	Restorative	D2000 – D2999
IV.	Endodontics	D3000 – D3999
V.	Periodontics	D4000 – D4999
VI.	Prosthodontics, removable	D5000 – D5899
VII.	Maxillofacial Prosthetics	D5900 – D5999
VIII.	Implant Services	D6000 – D6199
IX.	Prosthodontics, fixed	D6200 – D6999
X.	Oral & Maxillofacial Surgery	D7000 – D7999
XI.	Orthodontics	D8000 – D8999
XII.	Adjunctive General Services	D9000 – D9999

These categories exist solely as a means to organize the CDT Code. As a result, some categories of service are divided into subcategories of related procedures. Many categories and subcategories have descriptors applicable to all procedure codes therein.

Dental procedure codes within a Category of Service, or a subcategory, are not always in numeric order. The reason is that existing numeric sequences often do not have unassigned codes available for CDT Code additions.

Components of a Dental Procedure Code Entry

Every procedure in the CDT Code must have the first two of the following three components:

1. Procedure Code – A five character alphanumeric code beginning with the letter "D" that identifies a specific dental procedure. A Procedure Code cannot be changed or abbreviated.

2. Nomenclature – The written title of a Procedure Code. Nomenclature may be abbreviated when printed on claim forms or other documents that are subject to space limitation. Any such abbreviation does not constitute a change to the Nomenclature.

3. Descriptor – A written narrative that further defines the nature and intended use of a single Procedure Code, or group of such codes. A Descriptor, when present, follows the applicable Procedure Code and its Nomenclature. Descriptors that apply to a series of Procedure Codes precede that series of codes.

Using the CDT Code

The following points should prove helpful when using the CDT Code for recording services provided on the patient record, and when reporting procedures on a paper or electronic claim submission.

1. The presence of a CDT Code does not mean that the procedure is:
   a. endorsed by any entity or is considered a standard of care
   b. covered or reimbursed by a dental benefits plan

2. General practitioners, specialists, and other individuals may report any of the listed CDT Codes as long as they are acting within the scope of their state law.

3. CDT Codes that require inclusion of a narrative description on the claim have the words "by report" in their nomenclature.

4. "Unspecified... procedure, by report" codes are used when, in the opinion of the dentist, there is no other CDT Code entry that accurately describes the services provided the patient.

Required Statement

If there is more than one code in this edition that consists of a procedure and a dentist submits a claim under one of these codes, the payor may process the claim under any of these codes that is consistent with the payor's reimbursement policy.

1

Code on Dental Procedures and Nomenclature

Code on Dental Procedures and Nomenclature

The current version of the *Code on Dental Procedures and Nomenclature* (CDT Code) that follows is effective for the calendar year January 1, 2013 through December 31, 2013. There are a number of changes from the prior version, which are identified by the following symbols:

- New procedure code.
- ▲ Revision to a nomenclature or descriptor

Dental procedure codes that are no longer valid are not present. Chapter 2 contains the summary of all additions, revisions and deletions effective January 1, 2013.

As noted in the "Preface" the CDT Code is divided into twelve Categories of Service, and each category begins at the top of a right-hand page in this section of the manual.

Please note that when a code's nomenclature includes a "by report" notation, a narrative explaining the treatment provided must be included with the claim submission.

Classification of Materials

Names of dental materials are included in numerous procedure nomenclatures within several Categories of Service (e.g., Restorative; Prosthodontics, fixed). The following list of dental materials is included in the CDT Code *solely to aid to selection* of a procedure code applicable to the service provided.

Classification of Metals (Source: ADA Council on Scientific Affairs – online at: *ADA.org/2190.aspx*)

The noble metal classification system has been adopted as a more precise method of reporting various alloys used in dentistry. The alloys are defined on the basis of the percentage of metal content.

CLASSIFICATION	REQUIREMENT
High Noble Alloys	Noble Metal Content ≥ 60% (gold+ platinum group*) and gold ≥ 40%
Titanium and Titanium Alloys	Titanium ≥ 85%
Noble Alloys	Noble Metal Content ≥ 25% (gold + platinum group*)
Predominantly Base Alloys	Noble Metal Content < 25% (gold + platinum group*)

* metals of the platinum group are platinum, palladium, rhodium, iridium, osmium and ruthenium

▲ **Porcelain/ceramic**
Refers to pressed, fired, polished or milled materials containing predominantly inorganic refractory compounds including porcelains, glasses, ceramics, and glass-ceramics.

Resin
Refers to any resin-based composite, including fiber or ceramic reinforced polymer compounds.

● new procedure code   ▲ revision to a nomenclature or descriptor

D0100-D0999 I. Diagnostic

Clinical Oral Evaluations

The codes in this section recognize the cognitive skills necessary for patient evaluation. The collection and recording of some data and components of the dental examination may be delegated; however, the evaluation, which includes diagnosis and treatment planning, is the responsibility of the dentist. As with all ADA procedure codes, there is no distinction made between the evaluations provided by general practitioners and specialists. Report additional diagnostic and/or definitive procedures separately.

D0120 **periodic oral evaluation – established patient**
An evaluation performed on a patient of record to determine any changes in the patient's dental and medical health status since a previous comprehensive or periodic evaluation. This includes an oral cancer evaluation and periodontal screening where indicated, and may require interpretation of information acquired through additional diagnostic procedures. Report additional diagnostic procedures separately.

D0140 **limited oral evaluation – problem focused**
An evaluation limited to a specific oral health problem or complaint. This may require interpretation of information acquired through additional diagnostic procedures. Report additional diagnostic procedures separately. Definitive procedures may be required on the same date as the evaluation.

Typically, patients receiving this type of evaluation present with a specific problem and/or dental emergencies, trauma, acute infections, etc.

D0145 **oral evaluation for a patient under three years of age and counseling with primary caregiver**
Diagnostic services performed for a child under the age of three, preferably within the first six months of the eruption of the first primary tooth, including recording the oral and physical health history, evaluation of caries susceptibility, development of an appropriate preventive oral health regimen and communication with and counseling of the child's parent, legal guardian and/or primary caregiver.

D0150   comprehensive oral evaluation – new or established patient

Used by a general dentist and/or a specialist when evaluating a patient comprehensively. This applies to new patients; established patients who have had a significant change in health conditions or other unusual circumstances, by report, or established patients who have been absent from active treatment for three or more years. It is a thorough evaluation and recording of the extraoral and intraoral hard and soft tissues. It may require interpretation of information acquired through additional diagnostic procedures. Additional diagnostic procedures should be reported separately.

This includes an evaluation for oral cancer where indicated, the evaluation and recording of the patient's dental and medical history and a general health assessment. It may include the evaluation and recording of dental caries, missing or unerupted teeth, restorations, existing prostheses, occlusal relationships, periodontal conditions (including periodontal screening and/or charting), hard and soft tissue anomalies, etc.

D0160   detailed and extensive oral evaluation – problem focused, by report

A detailed and extensive problem focused evaluation entails extensive diagnostic and cognitive modalities based on the findings of a comprehensive oral evaluation. Integration of more extensive diagnostic modalities to develop a treatment plan for a specific problem is required. The condition requiring this type of evaluation should be described and documented.

Examples of conditions requiring this type of evaluation may include dentofacial anomalies, complicated perio-prosthetic conditions, complex temporomandibular dysfunction, facial pain of unknown origin, conditions requiring multi-disciplinary consultation, etc.

D0170   re-evaluation – limited, problem focused (established patient; not post-operative visit)

Assessing the status of a previously existing condition. For example:

- a traumatic injury where no treatment was rendered but patient needs follow-up monitoring;

- evaluation for undiagnosed continuing pain;

- soft tissue lesion requiring follow-up evaluation.

● new procedure code   ▲ revision to a nomenclature or descriptor

D0180 **comprehensive periodontal evaluation – new or established patient**

This procedure is indicated for patients showing signs or symptoms of periodontal disease and for patients with risk factors such as smoking or diabetes. It includes evaluation of periodontal conditions, probing and charting, evaluation and recording of the patient's dental and medical history and general health assessment. It may include the evaluation and recording of dental caries, missing or unerupted teeth, restorations, occlusal relationships and oral cancer evaluation.

• Pre-diagnostic Services

• D0190 **screening of a patient**

A screening, including state or federally mandated screenings, to determine an individual's need to be seen by a dentist for diagnosis.

• D0191 **assessment of a patient**

A limited clinical inspection that is performed to identify possible signs of oral or systemic disease, malformation, or injury, and the potential need for referral for diagnosis and treatment.

▲ Diagnostic Imaging

Should be taken only for clinical reasons as determined by the patient's dentist. Should be of diagnostic quality and properly identified and dated. Is a part of the patient's clinical record and the original images should be retained by the dentist. Originals should not be used to fulfill requests made by patients or third-parties for copies of records.

• Image Capture with Interpretation

▲ D0210 **intraoral – complete series of radiographic images**

A radiographic survey of the whole mouth, usually consisting of 14-22 periapical and posterior bitewing images intended to display the crowns and roots of all teeth, periapical areas and alveolar bone.

▲ D0220 **intraoral – periapical first radiographic image**

▲ D0230 **intraoral – periapical each additional radiographic image**

▲ D0240 **intraoral – occlusal radiographic image**

▲ **D0250 extraoral – first radiographic image**

▲ **D0260 extraoral – each additional radiographic image**

▲ **D0270 bitewing – single radiographic image**

▲ **D0272 bitewings – two radiographic images**

▲ **D0273 bitewings – three radiographic images**

▲ **D0274 bitewings – four radiographic images**

▲ **D0277 vertical bitewings – 7 to 8 radiographic images**
This does not constitute a full mouth intraoral radiographic series.

▲ **D0290 posterior-anterior or lateral skull and facial bone survey radiographic image**

D0310 sialography

D0320 temporomandibular joint arthrogram, including injection

▲ **D0321 other temporomandibular joint radiographic images, by report**

D0322 tomographic survey

▲ **D0330 panoramic radiographic image**

▲ **D0340 cephalometric radiographic image**

D0350 oral/facial photographic images
This includes photographic images, including those obtained by intraoral and extraoral cameras, excluding radiographic images. These photographic images should be a part of the patient's clinical record.

D0363 cone beam – three-dimensional image reconstruction using existing data, includes multiple images

● **D0364 cone beam CT capture and interpretation with limited field of view – less than one whole jaw**

● **D0365 cone beam CT capture and interpretation with field of view of one full dental arch – mandible**

● **D0366 cone beam CT capture and interpretation with field of view of one full dental arch – maxilla, with or without cranium**

Code on Dental Procedures and Nomenclature

- **D0367** cone beam CT capture and interpretation with field of view of both jaws; with or without cranium

- **D0368** cone beam CT capture and interpretation for TMJ series including two or more exposures

- **D0369** maxillofacial MRI capture and interpretation

- **D0370** maxillofacial ultrasound capture and interpretation

- **D0371** sialoendoscopy capture and interpretation

- **Image Capture Only**

  Interpretation and Report Performed by a Practitioner Not Associated With the Capture

- **D0380** cone beam CT image capture with limited field of view – less than one whole jaw

- **D0381** cone beam CT image capture with field of view of one full dental arch – mandible

- **D0382** cone beam CT image capture with field of view of one full dental arch – maxilla, with or without cranium

- **D0383** cone beam CT image capture with field of view of both jaws, with or without cranium

- **D0384** cone beam CT image capture for TMJ series including two or more exposures

- **D0385** maxillofacial MRI image capture

- **D0386** maxillofacial ultrasound image capture

- **Interpretation and Report Only**

  Image Capture Performed by a Practitioner Not Associated With Interpretation and Report

- **D0391** interpretation of diagnostic image by a practitioner not associated with capture of the image, including report

Tests and Examinations

D0415 **collection of microorganisms for culture and sensitivity**

D0416 **viral culture**
A diagnostic test to identify viral organisms, most often herpes virus.

D0417 **collection and preparation of saliva sample for laboratory diagnostic testing**

D0418 **analysis of saliva sample**
Chemical or biological analysis of saliva sample for diagnostic purposes.

D0421 **genetic test for susceptibility to oral diseases**
Sample collection for the purpose of certified laboratory analysis to detect specific genetic variations associated with increased susceptibility for oral diseases such as severe periodontal disease.

D0425 **caries susceptibility tests**
Not to be used for carious dentin staining.

D0431 **adjunctive pre-diagnostic test that aids in detection of mucosal abnormalities including premalignant and malignant lesions, not to include cytology or biopsy procedures**

D0460 **pulp vitality tests**
Includes multiple teeth and contra lateral comparison(s), as indicated.

D0470 **diagnostic casts**
Also known as diagnostic models or study models.

Oral Pathology Laboratory (Use Codes D0472 – D0502)

These are procedures generally performed in a pathology laboratory and do not include the removal of the tissue sample from the patient. For removal of tissue sample, see codes D7285 and D7286.

D0472 **accession of tissue, gross examination, preparation and transmission of written report**
To be used in reporting architecturally intact tissue obtained by invasive means.

D0473 **accession of tissue, gross and microscopic examination, preparation and transmission of written report**
To be used in reporting architecturally intact tissue obtained by invasive means.

D0474 **accession of tissue, gross and microscopic examination, including assessment of surgical margins for presence of disease, preparation and transmission of written report**
To be used in reporting architecturally intact tissue obtained by invasive means.

D0480 **accession of exfoliative cytologic smears, microscopic examination, preparation and transmission of written report**
To be used in reporting disaggregated, non-transepithelial cell cytology sample via mild scraping of the oral mucosa.

D0486 **laboratory accession of transepithelial cytologic sample, microscopic examination, preparation and transmission of written report**
Analysis, and written report of findings, of cytological sample of disaggregated transepithelial cells.

D0475 **decalcification procedure**
Procedure in which hard tissue is processed in order to allow sectioning and subsequent microscopic examination.

D0476 **special stains for microorganisms**
Procedure in which additional stains are applied to biopsy or surgical specimen in order to identify microorganisms.

D0477 **special stains, not for microorganisms**
Procedure in which additional stains are applied to a biopsy or surgical specimen in order to identify such things as melanin, mucin, iron, glycogen, etc.

D0478 **immunohistochemical stains**
A procedure in which specific antibody based reagents are applied to tissue samples in order to facilitate diagnosis.

D0479 **tissue in-situ hybridization, including interpretation**
A procedure which allows for the identification of nucleic acids, DNA and RNA, in the tissue sample in order to aid in the diagnosis of microorganisms and tumors.

D0481   electron microscopy – diagnostic
An extreme high magnification diagnostic procedure that enables identification of cell components and microorganisms that are otherwise not identifiable under light microscopy.

D0482   direct immunofluorescence
A technique used to identify immunoreactants which are localized to the patient's skin or mucous membranes.

D0483   indirect immunofluorescence
A technique used to identify circulating immunoreactants.

D0484   consultation on slides prepared elsewhere
A service provided in which microscopic slides of a biopsy specimen prepared at another laboratory are evaluated to aid in the diagnosis of a difficult case or to offer a consultative opinion at the patient's request. The findings are delivered by written report.

D0485   consultation, including preparation of slides from biopsy material supplied by referring source
A service that requires the consulting pathologist to prepare the slides as well as render a written report. The slides are evaluated to aid in the diagnosis of a difficult case or to offer a consultative opinion at the patient's request.

D0502   other oral pathology procedures, by report

D0999   unspecified diagnostic procedure, by report
Used for procedure that is not adequately described by a code. Describe procedure.

● new procedure code   ▲ revision to a nomenclature or descriptor

Code on Dental Procedures and Nomenclature

D1000–D1999   II. Preventive

Dental Prophylaxis

D1110   prophylaxis – adult
Removal of plaque, calculus and stains from the tooth structures in the permanent and transitional dentition. It is intended to control local irritational factors.

D1120   prophylaxis – child
Removal of plaque, calculus and stains from the tooth structures in the primary and transitional dentition. It is intended to control local irritational factors.

Topical Fluoride Treatment (Office Procedure)

Prescription strength fluoride product designed solely for use in the dental office, delivered to the dentition under the direct supervision of a dental professional. Fluoride must be applied separately from prophylaxis paste.

▲ **D1206   topical application of fluoride varnish**

● **D1208   topical application of fluoride**

Other Preventive Services

D1310   nutritional counseling for control of dental disease
Counseling on food selection and dietary habits as a part of treatment and control of periodontal disease and caries.

D1320   tobacco counseling for the control and prevention of oral disease
Tobacco prevention and cessation services reduce patient risks of developing tobacco-related oral diseases and conditions and improves prognosis for certain dental therapies.

D1330   oral hygiene instructions
This may include instructions for home care. Examples include tooth brushing technique, flossing, and use of special oral hygiene aids.

D1351 **sealant - per tooth**
Mechanically and/or chemically prepared enamel surface sealed to prevent decay.

D1352 **preventive resin restoration in a moderate to high caries risk patient – permanent tooth**
Conservative restoration of an active cavitated lesion in a pit or fissure that does not extend into dentin; includes placement of a sealant in any radiating non-carious fissures or pits.

Space Maintenance (Passive Appliances)

Passive appliances are designed to prevent tooth movement.

D1510 **space maintainer – fixed - unilateral**

D1515 **space maintainer – fixed - bilateral**

D1520 **space maintainer – removable – unilateral**

D1525 **space maintainer – removable – bilateral**

D1550 **re-cementation of space maintainer**

D1555 **removal of fixed space maintainer**
Procedure delivered by dentist who did not originally place the appliance, or by the practice where the appliance was originally delivered to the patient.

● new procedure code   ▲ revision to a nomenclature or descriptor

D2000–D2999   III. Restorative

Local anesthesia is usually considered to be part of Restorative procedures.

A one-surface posterior restoration is one in which the restoration involves only one of the five surface classifications (mesial, distal, occlusal, lingual, or facial, including buccal and labial).

A two-surface posterior restoration is one in which the restoration extends to two of the five surface classifications.

A three-surface posterior restoration is one in which the restoration extends to three of the five surface classifications.

A four-or-more surface posterior restoration is one in which the restoration extends to four or more of the five surface classifications.

A one-surface anterior proximal restoration is one in which neither the lingual nor the facial margins of the restoration extend beyond the line angle.

A two-surface anterior proximal restoration is one in which either the lingual or facial margin of the restoration extends beyond the line angle.

A three-surface anterior proximal restoration is one in which both the lingual and facial margins of the restorations extend beyond the line angle.

A four-or-more surface anterior restoration is one in which both the lingual and facial margins extend beyond the line angle and the incisal angle is involved. This restoration might also involve all four surfaces of an anterior tooth and not involve the incisal angle.

Amalgam Restorations (Including Polishing)

Tooth preparation, all adhesives (including amalgam bonding agents), liners and bases are included as part of the restoration. If pins are used, they should be reported separately (see D2951).

D2140   amalgam – one surface, primary or permanent

D2150   amalgam – two surfaces, primary or permanent

D2160   amalgam – three surfaces, primary or permanent

D2161   amalgam – four or more surfaces, primary or permanent

Resin-Based Composite Restorations – Direct

Resin-based composite refers to a broad category of materials including but not limited to composites. May include bonded composite, light-cured composite, etc. Tooth preparation, acid etching, adhesives (including resin bonding agents), liners and bases and curing are included as part of the restoration. Glass ionomers, when used as restorations, should be reported with these codes. If pins are used, they should be reported separately (see D2951).

D2330 resin-based composite – one surface, anterior

D2331 resin-based composite – two surfaces, anterior

D2332 resin-based composite – three surfaces, anterior

D2335 resin-based composite – four or more surfaces or involving incisal angle (anterior)
Incisal angle to be defined as one of the angles formed by the junction of the incisal and the mesial or distal surface of an anterior tooth.

D2390 resin-based composite crown, anterior
Full resin-based composite coverage of tooth.

D2391 resin-based composite – one surface, posterior
Used to restore a carious lesion into the dentin or a deeply eroded area into the dentin. Not a preventive procedure.

D2392 resin-based composite – two surfaces, posterior

D2393 resin-based composite – three surfaces, posterior

D2394 resin-based composite – four or more surfaces, posterior

Gold Foil Restorations

D2410 gold foil – one surface

D2420 gold foil – two surfaces

D2430 gold foil – three surfaces

1

Code on Dental Procedures and Nomenclature

Inlay/Onlay Restorations

D2510 inlay – metallic – one surface

D2520 inlay – metallic – two surfaces

D2530 inlay – metallic – three or more surfaces

D2542 onlay – metallic – two surfaces

D2543 onlay – metallic – three surfaces

D2544 onlay – metallic – four or more surfaces
Porcelain/ceramic inlays/onlays include all indirect ceramic and porcelain type inlays/onlays.

D2610 inlay – porcelain/ceramic – one surface

D2620 inlay – porcelain/ceramic – two surfaces

D2630 inlay – porcelain/ceramic – three or more surfaces

D2642 onlay – porcelain/ceramic – two surfaces

D2643 onlay – porcelain/ceramic – three surfaces

D2644 onlay – porcelain/ceramic – four or more surfaces
Resin-based composite inlays/onlays must utilize indirect technique.

D2650 inlay – resin-based composite – one surface

D2651 inlay – resin-based composite – two surfaces

D2652 inlay – resin-based composite – three or more surfaces

D2662 onlay – resin-based composite – two surfaces

D2663 onlay – resin-based composite – three surfaces

D2664 onlay – resin-based composite – four or more surfaces

Crowns - Single Restorations Only

▲ **D2710 crown – resin-based composite (indirect)**

D2712 crown – ¾ resin-based composite (indirect)
This code does not include facial veneers.

D2720 crown – resin with high noble metal

D2721 crown – resin with predominantly base metal

D2722 crown – resin with noble metal

D2740 crown – porcelain/ceramic substrate

D2750 crown – porcelain fused to high noble metal

D2751 crown – porcelain fused to predominantly base metal

D2752 crown – porcelain fused to noble metal

D2780 crown – ¾ cast high noble metal

D2781 crown – ¾ cast predominantly base metal

D2782 crown – ¾ cast noble metal

D2783 crown – ¾ porcelain/ceramic
This code does not include facial veneers.

D2790 crown – full cast high noble metal

D2791 crown – full cast predominantly base metal

D2792 crown – full cast noble metal

D2794 crown – titanium

▲ **D2799 provisional crown– further treatment or completion
of diagnosis necessary prior to final impression**
Not to be used as a temporary crown for a routine
prosthetic restoration.

Other Restorative Services

- **D2990   resin infiltration of incipient smooth surface lesions**
  Placement of an infiltrating resin restoration for strengthening, stabilizing and/or limiting the progression of the lesion.

  D2910   recement inlay, onlay, or partial coverage restoration

  D2915   recement cast or prefabricated post and core

  D2920   recement crown

- **D2929   prefabricated porcelain/ceramic crown – primary tooth**

  D2930   prefabricated stainless steel crown – primary tooth

  D2931   prefabricated stainless steel crown – permanent tooth

  D2932   prefabricated resin crown

  D2933   prefabricated stainless steel crown with resin window
  Open-face stainless steel crown with aesthetic resin facing or veneer.

  D2934   prefabricated esthetic coated stainless steel crown – primary tooth
  Stainless steel primary crown with exterior esthetic coating.

▲ **D2940   protective restoration**
  Direct placement of a restorative material to protect tooth and/or tissue form. This procedure may be used to relieve pain, promote healing, or prevent further deterioration. Not to be used for endodontic access closure, or as a base or liner under restoration.

  D2950   core buildup, including any pins
  Refers to building up of anatomical crown when restorative crown will be placed, whether or not pins are used. A material is placed in the tooth preparation for a crown when there is insufficient tooth strength and retention for the crown procedure. This should not be reported when the procedure only involves a filler to eliminate any undercut, box form, or concave irregularity in the preparation.

  D2951   pin retention – per tooth, in addition to restoration

D2952 post and core in addition to crown, indirectly fabricated
Post and core are custom fabricated as a single unit.

D2953 each additional indirectly fabricated post – same tooth
To be used with D2952.

D2954 prefabricated post and core in addition to crown
Core is built around a prefabricated post. This procedure includes the core material.

▲ **D2955 post removal**

D2957 each additional prefabricated post – same tooth
To be used with D2954.

D2960 labial veneer (resin laminate) – chairside
Refers to labial/facial direct resin bonded veneers.

D2961 labial veneer (resin laminate) – laboratory
Refers to labial/facial indirect resin bonded veneers.

D2962 labial veneer (porcelain laminate) – laboratory
Refers also to facial veneers that extend interproximally and/or cover the incisal edge. Porcelain/ceramic veneers presently include all ceramic and porcelain veneers.

D2970 temporary crown (fractured tooth)
Usually a preformed artificial crown, which is fitted over a damaged tooth as an immediate protective device. This is not to be used as temporization during crown fabrication.

D2971 additional procedures to construct new crown under existing partial denture framework
To be reported in addition to a crown code.

D2975 coping
A thin covering of the remaining portion of a tooth, usually fabricated of metal and devoid of anatomic contour. This is to be used as a definitive restoration.

▲ **D2980   crown repair necessitated by restorative material failure**

● **D2981   inlay repair necessitated by restorative material failure**

● **D2982   onlay repair necessitated by restorative material failure**

● **D2983   veneer repair necessitated by restorative material failure**

D2999   unspecified restorative procedure, by report
Use for procedure that is not adequately described by a code.
Describe procedure.

D3000–D3999   IV. Endodontics

Local anesthesia is usually considered to be part of Endodontic procedures.

Pulp Capping

D3110   pulp cap – direct (excluding final restoration)
Procedure in which the exposed pulp is covered with a dressing or cement that protects the pulp and promotes healing and repair.

D3120   pulp cap – indirect (excluding final restoration)
Procedure in which the nearly exposed pulp is covered with a protective dressing to protect the pulp from additional injury and to promote healing and repair via formation of secondary dentin. This code is not to be used for bases and liners when all caries has been removed.

Pulpotomy

D3220   therapeutic pulpotomy (excluding final restoration) – removal of pulp coronal to the dentinocemental junction and application of medicament
Pulpotomy is the surgical removal of a portion of the pulp with the aim of maintaining the vitality of the remaining portion by means of an adequate dressing.

– To be performed on primary or permanent teeth.

– This is not to be construed as the first stage of root canal therapy.

– Not to be used for apexogenesis.

D3221   pulpal debridement, primary and permanent teeth
Pulpal debridement for the relief of acute pain prior to conventional root canal therapy. This procedure is not to be used when endodontic treatment is completed on the same day.

D3222 **partial pulpotomy for apexogenesis – permanent tooth with incomplete root development**
Removal of a portion of the pulp and application of a medicament with the aim of maintaining the vitality of the remaining portion to encourage continued physiological development and formation of the root. This procedure is not to be construed as the first stage of root canal therapy.

Endodontic Therapy on Primary Teeth

Endodontic therapy on primary teeth with succedaneous teeth and placement of resorbable filling. This includes pulpectomy, cleaning, and filling of canals with resorbable material.

D3230 **pulpal therapy (resorbable filling) – anterior, primary tooth (excluding final restoration)**
Primary incisors and cuspids.

D3240 **pulpal therapy (resorbable filling) – posterior, primary tooth (excluding final restoration)**
Primary first and second molars.

Endodontic Therapy (Including Treatment Plan, Clinical Procedures and Follow-Up Care)

Includes primary teeth without succedaneous teeth and permanent teeth. Complete root canal therapy; pulpectomy is part of root canal therapy.

Includes all appointments necessary to complete treatment; also includes intra-operative radiographs. Does not include diagnostic evaluation and necessary radiographs/diagnostic images.

D3310 **endodontic therapy, anterior tooth (excluding final restoration)**

D3320 **endodontic therapy, bicuspid tooth (excluding final restoration)**

D3330 **endodontic therapy, molar (excluding final restoration)**

● new procedure code   ▲ revision to a nomenclature or descriptor

D3331 **treatment of root canal obstruction; non-surgical access**
In lieu of surgery, the formation of a pathway to achieve an apical seal without surgical intervention because of a non-negotiable root canal blocked by foreign bodies, including but not limited to separated instruments, broken posts or calcification of 50% or more of the length of the tooth root.

D3332 **incomplete endodontic therapy; inoperable, unrestorable or fractured tooth**
Considerable time is necessary to determine diagnosis and/or provide initial treatment before the fracture makes the tooth unretainable.

D3333 **internal root repair of perforation defects**
Non-surgical seal of perforation caused by resorption and/or decay but not iatrogenic by provider filing claim.

▲ **Endodontic Retreatment**

D3346 **retreatment of previous root canal therapy – anterior**

D3347 **retreatment of previous root canal therapy – bicuspid**

D3348 **retreatment of previous root canal therapy – molar**
Apexification/Recalcification and Pulpal Regeneration Procedures

D3351 **apexification/recalcification/pulpal regeneration – initial visit (apical closure/calcific repair of perforations, root resorption, pulp space disinfection, etc.)**
Includes opening tooth, preparation of canal spaces, first placement of medication and necessary radiographs. (This procedure may include first phase of complete root canal therapy.)

▲ **D3352** **apexification/recalcification/pulpal regeneration – interim medication replacement**
For visits in which the intra-canal medication is replaced with new medication. Includes any necessary radiographs.

D3353 **apexification/recalcification – final visit (includes completed root canal therapy – apical closure/calcific repair of perforations, root resorption, etc.)**
Includes removal of intra-canal medication and procedures necessary to place final root canal filling material including necessary radiographs. (This procedure includes last phase of complete root canal therapy.)

D3354 **pulpal regeneration – (completion of regenerative treatment in an immature permanent tooth with a necrotic pulp); does not include final restoration**
Includes removal of intra-canal medication and procedures necessary to regenerate continued root development and necessary radiographs. This procedure includes placement of a seal at the coronal portion of the root canal system. Conventional root canal treatment is not performed.

Apicoectomy/Periradicular Services

Periradicular surgery is a term used to describe surgery to the root surface (e.g., apicoectomy), repair of a root perforation or resorptive defect, exploratory curettage to look for root fractures, removal of extruded filling materials or instruments, removal of broken root fragments, sealing of accessory canals, etc. This does not include retrograde filling material placement.

D3410 **apicoectomy/periradicular surgery – anterior**
For surgery on root of anterior tooth. Does not include placement of retrograde filling material.

D3421 **apicoectomy/periradicular surgery – bicuspid (first root)**
For surgery on one root of a bicuspid. Does not include placement of retrograde filling material. If more than one root is treated, see D3426.

D3425 **apicoectomy/periradicular surgery – molar (first root)**
For surgery on one root of a molar tooth. Does not include placement of retrograde filling material. If more than one root is treated, see D3426.

● new procedure code   ▲ revision to a nomenclature or descriptor

D3426 **apicoectomy/periradicular surgery (each additional root)**
Typically used for bicuspids and molar surgeries when more than one root is treated during the same procedure. This does not include retrograde filling material placement.

D3430 **retrograde filling – per root**
For placement of retrograde filling material during periradicular surgery procedures. If more than one filling is placed in one root report as D3999 and describe.

D3450 **root amputation – per root**
Root resection of a multi-rooted tooth while leaving the crown. If the crown is sectioned, see D3920.

D3460 **endodontic endosseous implant**
Placement of implant material, which extends from a pulpal space into the bone beyond the end of the root.

D3470 **intentional reimplantation (including necessary splinting)**
For the intentional removal, inspection and treatment of the root and replacement of a tooth into its own socket. This does not include necessary retrograde filling material placement.

Other Endodontic Procedures

D3910 **surgical procedure for isolation of tooth with rubber dam**

D3920 **hemisection (including any root removal), not including root canal therapy**
Includes separation of a multi-rooted tooth into separate sections containing the root and the overlying portion of the crown. It may also include the removal of one or more of those sections.

D3950 **canal preparation and fitting of preformed dowel or post**
Should not be reported in conjunction with D2952, D2953, D2954 or D2957 by the same practitioner.

D3999 **unspecified endodontic procedure, by report**
Used for procedure that is not adequately described by a code. Describe procedure.

D4000-D4999 V. Periodontics

Local anesthesia is usually considered to be part of Periodontal procedures.

Surgical Services (Including Usual Postoperative Care)

Site: A term used to describe a single area, position, or locus. The word "site" is frequently used to indicate an area of soft tissue recession on a single tooth or an osseous defect adjacent to a single tooth; also used to indicate soft tissue defects and/or osseous defects in edentulous tooth positions.

– If two contiguous teeth have areas of soft tissue recession, each area of recession is a single site.

– If two contiguous teeth have adjacent but separate osseous defects, each defect is a single site.

– If two contiguous teeth have a communicating interproximal osseous defect, it should be considered a single site.

– All non-communicating osseous defects are single sites.

– All edentulous non-contiguous tooth positions are single sites.

– Depending on the dimensions of the defect, up to two contiguous edentulous tooth positions may be considered a single site.

Tooth Bounded Space: A space created by one or more missing teeth that has a tooth on each side.

▲ **D4210** **gingivectomy or gingivoplasty – four or more contiguous teeth or tooth bounded spaces per quadrant**
It is performed to eliminate suprabony pockets or to restore normal architecture when gingival enlargements or asymmetrical or unaesthetic topography is evident with normal bony configuration.

▲ **D4211** **gingivectomy or gingivoplasty – one to three contiguous teeth or tooth bounded spaces per quadrant**
It is performed to eliminate suprabony pockets or to restore normal architecture when gingival enlargements or asymmetrical or unaesthetic topography is evident with normal bony configuration.

- **D4212** **gingivectomy or gingivoplasty to allow access for restorative procedure, per tooth**

  D4230 **anatomical crown exposure – four or more contiguous teeth per quadrant**
  This procedure is utilized in an otherwise periodontally healthy area to remove enlarged gingival tissue and supporting bone (ostectomy) to provide an anatomically correct gingival relationship.

  D4231 **anatomical crown exposure – one to three teeth per quadrant**
  This procedure is utilized in an otherwise periodontally healthy area to remove enlarged gingival tissue and supporting bone (ostectomy) to provide an anatomically correct gingival relationship.

  D4240 **gingival flap procedure, including root planing – four or more contiguous teeth or tooth bounded spaces per quadrant**
  A soft tissue flap is reflected or resected to allow debridement of the root surface and the removal of granulation tissue. Osseous recontouring is not accomplished in conjunction with this procedure. May include open flap curettage, reverse bevel flap surgery, modified Kirkland flap procedure, and modified Widman surgery. This procedure is performed in the presence of moderate to deep probing depths, loss of attachment, need to maintain esthetics, need for increased access to the root surface and alveolar bone, or to determine the presence of a cracked tooth, fractured root, or external root resorption. Other procedures may be required concurrent to D4240 and should be reported separately using their own unique codes.

  D4241 **gingival flap procedure, including root planing – one to three contiguous teeth or tooth bounded spaces per quadrant**
  A soft tissue flap is reflected or resected to allow debridement of the root surface and the removal of granulation tissue. Osseous recontouring is not accomplished in conjunction with this procedure. May include open flap curettage, reverse bevel flap surgery, modified Kirkland flap procedure, and modified Widman surgery. This procedure is performed in the presence of moderate to deep probing depths, loss of attachment, need to maintain esthetics, need for increased access to the root surface and alveolar bone, or to determine the presence of a cracked tooth, fractured root, or external root resorption. Other procedures may be required concurrent to D4241 and should be reported separately using their own unique codes.

● new procedure code   ▲ revision to a nomenclature or descriptor

D4245 apically positioned flap
Procedure is used to preserve keratinized gingiva in conjunction with osseous resection and second stage implant procedure. Procedure may also be used to preserve keratinized/attached gingiva during surgical exposure of labially impacted teeth, and may be used during treatment of peri-implantitis.

D4249 clinical crown lengthening – hard tissue
This procedure is employed to allow restorative procedure or crown with little or no tooth structure exposed to the oral cavity. Crown lengthening requires reflection of a flap and is performed in a healthy periodontal environment, as opposed to osseous surgery, which is performed in the presence of periodontal disease. Where there are adjacent teeth, the flap design may involve a larger surgical area.

▲ **D4260 osseous surgery (including flap entry and closure) – four or more contiguous teeth or tooth bounded spaces per quadrant**
This procedure modifies the bony support of the teeth by reshaping the alveolar process to achieve a more physiologic form. This must include the removal of supporting bone (ostectomy) and/or non-supporting bone (osteoplasty). Other procedures may be required concurrent to D4260 and should be reported using their own unique codes.

▲ **D4261 osseous surgery (including flap entry and closure) – one to three contiguous teeth or tooth bounded spaces per quadrant**
This procedure modifies the bony support of the teeth by reshaping the alveolar process to achieve a more physiologic form. This must include the removal of supporting bone (ostectomy) and/or non-supporting bone (osteoplasty). Other procedures may be required concurrent to D4261 and should be reported using their own unique codes.

D4263 bone replacement graft – first site in quadrant
This procedure involves the use of osseous autografts, osseous allografts, or non-osseous grafts to stimulate periodontal regeneration when the disease process has led to a deformity of the bone. This procedure does not include flap entry and closure, wound debridement, osseous contouring, or the placement of biologic materials to aid in osseous tissue regeneration or barrier membranes. Other separate procedures may be required concurrent to D4263 and should be reported using their own unique codes.

D4264 **bone replacement graft – each additional site in quadrant**
This procedure involves the use of osseous autografts, osseous allografts, or non-osseous grafts to stimulate periodontal regeneration when the disease process has led to a deformity of the bone. This procedure does not include flap entry and closure, wound debridement, osseous contouring, or the placement of biologic materials to aid in osseous tissue regeneration or barrier membranes. This code is used if performed concurrently with D4263 and allows reporting of the exact number of sites involved.

D4265 **biologic materials to aid in soft and osseous tissue regeneration**
Biologic materials may be used alone or with other regenerative substrates such as bone and barrier membranes, depending upon their formulation and the presentation of the periodontal defect. This procedure does not include surgical entry and closure, wound debridement, osseous contouring, or the placement of graft materials and/or barrier membranes. Other separate procedures may be required concurrent to D4265 and should be reported using their own unique codes.

▲ **D4266** **guided tissue regeneration – resorbable barrier, per site**
This procedure does not include flap entry and closure, or, when indicated, wound debridement, osseous contouring, bone replacement grafts, and placement of biologic materials to aid in osseous regeneration. This procedure can be used for periodontal and peri-implant defects.

▲ **D4267** **guided tissue regeneration – non-resorbable barrier, per site (includes membrane removal)**
This procedure does not include flap entry and closure, or, when indicated, wound debridement, osseous contouring, bone replacement grafts, and placement of biologic materials to aid in osseous regeneration. This procedure can be used for periodontal and peri-implant defects.

D4268 **surgical revision procedure, per tooth**
This procedure is to refine the results of a previously provided surgical procedure. This may require a surgical procedure to modify the irregular contours of hard or soft tissue. A mucoperiosteal flap may be elevated to allow access to reshape alveolar bone. The flaps are replaced or repositioned and sutured.

D4270 pedicle soft tissue graft procedure
A pedicle flap of gingiva can be raised from an edentulous ridge, adjacent teeth, or from the existing gingiva on the tooth and moved laterally or coronally to replace alveolar mucosa as marginal tissue. The procedure can be used to cover an exposed root or to eliminate a gingival defect if the root is not too prominent in the arch.

D4273 subepithelial connective tissue graft procedures, per tooth
This procedure is performed to create or augment gingiva, to obtain root coverage to eliminate sensitivity and to prevent root caries, to eliminate frenum pull, to extend the vestibular fornix, to augment collapsed ridges, to provide an adequate gingival interface with a restoration or to cover bone or ridge regeneration sites when adequate gingival tissues are not available for effective closure. There are two surgical sites. The recipient site utilizes a split thickness incision, retaining the overlying flap of gingiva and/ or mucosa. The connective tissue is dissected from the donor site leaving an epithelialized flap for closure. After the graft is placed on the recipient site, it is covered with the retained overlying flap.

D4274 distal or proximal wedge procedure (when not performed in conjunction with surgical procedures in the same anatomical area)
This procedure is performed in an edentulous area adjacent to a periodontally involved tooth. Gingival incisions are utilized to allow removal of a tissue wedge to gain access and correct the underlying osseous defect and to permit close flap adaptation.

D4275 soft tissue allograft
Procedure is performed to create or augment the gingiva, with or without root coverage. This may be used to eliminate the pull of the frena and muscle attachments, to extend the vestibular fornix, and correct localized gingival recession. There is no donor site.

D4276 combined connective tissue and double pedicle graft, per tooth
Advanced gingival recession often cannot be corrected with a single procedure. Combined tissue grafting procedures are needed to achieve the desired outcome.

● **D4277 free soft tissue graft procedure (including donor site surgery), first tooth or edentulous tooth position in graft**

● **D4278   free soft tissue graft procedure (including donor site surgery), each additional contiguous tooth or edentulous tooth position in same graft site**

Non-Surgical Periodontal Service

D4320   provisional splinting – intracoronal
This is an interim stabilization of mobile teeth. A variety of methods and appliances may be employed for this purpose. Identify the teeth involved.

D4321   provisional splinting – extracoronal
This is an interim stabilization of mobile teeth. A variety of methods and appliances may be employed for this purpose. Identify the teeth involved.

D4341   periodontal scaling and root planing – four or more teeth per quadrant
This procedure involves instrumentation of the crown and root surfaces of the teeth to remove plaque and calculus from these surfaces. It is indicated for patients with periodontal disease and is therapeutic, not prophylactic, in nature. Root planing is the definitive procedure designed for the removal of cementum and dentin that is rough, and/or permeated by calculus or contaminated with toxins or microorganisms. Some soft tissue removal occurs. This procedure may be used as a definitive treatment in some stages of periodontal disease and/or as a part of pre-surgical procedures in others.

D4342   periodontal scaling and root planing – one to three teeth per quadrant
This procedure involves instrumentation of the crown and root surfaces of the teeth to remove plaque and calculus from these surfaces. It is indicated for patients with periodontal disease and is therapeutic, not prophylactic, in nature. Root planing is the definitive procedure designed for the removal of cementum and dentin that is rough, and/or permeated by calculus or contaminated with toxins or microorganisms. Some soft tissue removal occurs. This procedure may be used as a definitive treatment in some stages of periodontal disease and/or as a part of pre-surgical procedures in others.

D4355 full mouth debridement to enable comprehensive evaluation and diagnosis

The gross removal of plaque and calculus that interfere with the ability of the dentist to perform a comprehensive oral evaluation. This preliminary procedure does not preclude the need for additional procedures.

▲ **D4381 localized delivery of antimicrobial agents via a controlled release vehicle into diseased crevicular tissue, per tooth**

FDA approved subgingival delivery devices containing antimicrobial medication(s) are inserted into periodontal pockets to suppress the pathogenic microbiota. These devices slowly release the pharmacological agents so they can remain at the intended site of action in a therapeutic concentration for a sufficient length of time.

Other Periodontal Services

D4910 periodontal maintenance

This procedure is instituted following periodontal therapy and continues at varying intervals, determined by the clinical evaluation of the dentist, for the life of the dentition or any implant replacements. It includes removal of the bacterial plaque and calculus from supragingival and subgingival regions, site specific scaling and root planing where indicated, and polishing the teeth. If new or recurring periodontal disease appears, additional diagnostic and treatment procedures must be considered.

D4920 unscheduled dressing change (by someone other than treating dentist)

D4999 unspecified periodontal procedure, by report

Use for procedure that is not adequately described by a code. Describe procedure.

D5000-D5899 VI. Prosthodontics (removable)

Local anesthesia is usually considered to be part of Removable Prosthodontic procedures.

Complete Dentures (Including Routine Post-Delivery Care)

D5110 complete denture – maxillary

D5120 complete denture – mandibular

D5130 immediate denture – maxillary
Includes limited follow-up care only; does not include required future rebasing/relining procedure(s) or a complete new denture.

D5140 immediate denture – mandibular
Includes limited follow-up care only; does not include required future rebasing/relining procedure(s) or a complete new denture.

Partial Dentures (Including Routine Post-Delivery Care)

D5211 maxillary partial denture – resin base (including any conventional clasps, rests and teeth)
Includes acrylic resin base denture with resin or wrought wire clasps.

D5212 mandibular partial denture – resin base (including any conventional clasps, rests and teeth)
Includes acrylic resin base denture with resin or wrought wire clasps.

D5213 maxillary partial denture – cast metal framework with resin denture bases (including any conventional clasps, rests and teeth)

D5214 mandibular partial denture – cast metal framework with resin denture bases (including any conventional clasps, rests and teeth)

D5225 maxillary partial denture – flexible base (including any clasps, rests and teeth)

D5226   mandibular partial denture – flexible base (including any clasps, rests and teeth)

D5281   removable unilateral partial denture – one piece cast metal (including clasps and teeth

Adjustments to Dentures

D5410   adjust complete denture – maxillary

D5411   adjust complete denture – mandibular

D5421   adjust partial denture – maxillary

D5422   adjust partial denture – mandibular

Repairs to Complete Dentures

D5510   repair broken complete denture base

D5520   replace missing or broken teeth – complete denture (each tooth)

Repairs to Partial Dentures

D5610   repair resin denture base

D5620   repair cast framework

D5630   repair or replace broken clasp

D5640   replace broken teeth - per tooth

D5650   add tooth to existing partial denture

D5660   add clasp to existing partial denture

D5670   replace all teeth and acrylic on cast metal framework (maxillary)

D5671   replace all teeth and acrylic on cast metal framework (mandibular)

Denture Rebase Procedures

Rebase – process of refitting a denture by replacing the base material.

D5710 **rebase complete maxillary denture**

D5711 **rebase complete mandibular denture**

D5720 **rebase maxillary partial denture**

D5721 **rebase mandibular partial denture**

Denture Reline Procedures

Reline is the process of resurfacing the tissue side of a denture with new base material.

D5730 **reline complete maxillary denture (chairside)**

D5731 **reline complete mandibular denture (chairside)**

D5740 **reline maxillary partial denture (chairside)**

D5741 **reline mandibular partial denture (chairside)**

D5750 **reline complete maxillary denture (laboratory)**

D5751 **reline complete mandibular denture (laboratory)**

D5760 **reline maxillary partial denture (laboratory)**

D5761 **reline mandibular partial denture (laboratory)**

Interim Prosthesis

A provisional prosthesis designed for use over a limited period of time, after which it is to be replaced by a more definitive restoration.

D5810 **interim complete denture (maxillary)**

D5811 **interim complete denture (mandibular)**

D5820 **interim partial denture (maxillary)**
Includes any necessary clasps and rests.

D5821 **interim partial denture (mandibular)**
Includes any necessary clasps and rests.

Other Removable Prosthetic Services

D5850 **tissue conditioning, maxillary**
Treatment reline using materials designed to heal unhealthy ridges prior to more definitive final restoration.

D5851 **tissue conditioning, mandibular**
Treatment reline using materials designed to heal unhealthy ridges prior to more definitive final restoration.

D5860 **overdenture – complete, by report**
Describe and document procedures as performed. Other separate procedures may be required concurrent to D5860.

D5861 **overdenture – partial, by report**
Describe and document procedures as performed. Other separate procedures may be required concurrent to D5861.

D5862 **precision attachment, by report**
Each set of male and female components should be reported as one precision attachment. Describe the type of attachment used.

D5867 **replacement of replaceable part of semi-precision or precision attachment (male or female component)**

D5875 **modification of removable prosthesis following implant surgery**
The modification of existing removable prosthesis is sometimes necessary at the time of implant placement and bone graft surgery and is always necessary at the time of the placement of the healing caps. This code could also be used to report the modification of an existing prosthesis when the abutments are placed and retentive elements are placed into the removable prosthesis, thereby reducing the need for a new prosthesis.

D5899 **unspecified removable prosthodontic procedure, by report**
Use for a procedure that is not adequately described by a code. Describe procedure.

D5900-D5999 VII. Maxillofacial Prosthetics

D5911 facial moulage (sectional)
A sectional facial moulage impression is a procedure used to record the soft tissue contours of a portion of the face. Occasionally several separate sectional impressions are made, and then reassembled to provide a full facial contour cast. The impression is utilized to create a partial facial moulage and generally is not reusable.

D5912 facial moulage (complete)
Synonymous terminology: facial impression, face mask impression.

A complete facial moulage impression is a procedure used to record the soft tissue contours of the whole face. The impression is utilized to create a facial moulage and generally is not reusable.

D5913 nasal prosthesis
Synonymous terminology: artificial nose.

A removable prosthesis attached to the skin, which artificially restores part or all of the nose. Fabrication of a nasal prosthesis requires creation of an original mold. Additional prostheses usually can be made from the same mold, and assuming no further tissue changes occur, the same mold can be utilized for extended periods of time.

When a new prosthesis is made from the existing mold, this procedure is termed a nasal prosthesis replacement.

D5914 auricular prosthesis
Synonymous terminology: artificial ear, ear prosthesis.

A removable prosthesis, which artificially restores part or all of the natural ear. Usually, replacement prostheses can be made from the original mold if tissue bed changes have not occurred. Creation of an auricular prosthesis requires fabrication of a mold, from which additional prostheses usually can be made, as needed later (auricular prosthesis, replacement).

Code on Dental Procedures and Nomenclature

D5915 orbital prosthesis

A prosthesis, which artificially restores the eye, eyelids, and adjacent hard and soft tissue, lost as a result of trauma or surgery.

Fabrication of an orbital prosthesis requires creation of an original mold. Additional prostheses usually can be made from the same mold, and assuming no further tissue changes occur, the same mold can be utilized for extended periods of time.

When a new prosthesis is made from the existing mold, this procedure is termed an orbital prosthesis replacement.

D5916 ocular prosthesis

Synonymous terminology: artificial eye, glass eye.

A prosthesis, which artificially replaces an eye missing as a result of trauma, surgery or congenital absence. The prosthesis does not replace missing eyelids or adjacent skin, mucosa or muscle.

Ocular prostheses require semiannual or annual cleaning and polishing. Also, occasional revisions to re-adapt the prosthesis to the tissue bed may be necessary. Glass eyes are rarely made and cannot be re-adapted.

D5919 facial prosthesis

Synonymous terminology: prosthetic dressing.

A removable prosthesis, which artificially replaces a portion of the face, lost due to surgery, trauma or congenital absence.

Flexion of natural tissues may preclude adaptation and movement of the prosthesis to match the adjacent skin. Salivary leakage, when communicating with the oral cavity, adversely affects retention.

D5922 nasal septal prosthesis

Synonymous terminology: Septal plug, septal button.

Removable prosthesis to occlude (obturate) a hole within the nasal septal wall. Adverse chemical degradation in this moist environment may require frequent replacement. Silicone prostheses are occasionally subject to fungal invasion.

D5923 ocular prosthesis, interim

Synonymous terminology: Eye shell, shell, ocular conformer, conformer.

A temporary replacement generally made of clear acrylic resin for an eye lost due to surgery or trauma. No attempt is made to re-establish esthetics. Fabrication of an interim ocular prosthesis generally implies subsequent fabrication of an aesthetic ocular prosthesis.

D5924 cranial prosthesis

Synonymous terminology: Skull plate, cranioplasty prosthesis, cranial implant.

A biocompatible, permanently implanted replacement of a portion of the skull bones; an artificial replacement for a portion of the skull bone.

D5925 facial augmentation implant prosthesis

Synonymous terminology: facial implant.

An implantable biocompatible material generally onlayed upon an existing bony area beneath the skin tissue to fill in or collectively raise portions of the overlaying facial skin tissues to create acceptable contours.

Although some forms of pre-made surgical implants are commercially available, the facial augmentation is usually custom made for surgical implantation for each individual patient due to the irregular or extensive nature of the facial deficit.

D5926 nasal prosthesis, replacement

Synonymous terminology: replacement nose.

An artificial nose produced from a previously made mold. A replacement prosthesis does not require fabrication of a new mold. Generally, several prostheses can be made from the same mold assuming no changes occur in the tissue bed due to surgery or age related topographical variations.

D5927 auricular prosthesis, replacement

Synonymous terminology: replacement ear.

An artificial ear produced from a previously made mold. A replacement prosthesis does not require fabrication of a new mold. Generally, several prostheses can be made from the same mold assuming no changes occur in the tissue bed due to surgery or age related topographical variations.

D5928   orbital prosthesis, replacement

A replacement for a previously made orbital prosthesis. A replacement prosthesis does not require fabrication of a new mold. Generally, several prostheses can be made from the same mold assuming no changes occur in the tissue bed due to surgery or age related topographical variations.

D5929   facial prosthesis, replacement

A replacement facial prosthesis made from the original mold. A replacement prosthesis does not require fabrication of a new mold. Generally, several prostheses can be made from the same mold assuming no changes occur in the tissue bed due to further surgery or age related topographical variations.

D5931   obturator prosthesis, surgical

Synonymous terminology: Obturator, surgical stayplate, immediate temporary obturator.

A temporary prosthesis inserted during or immediately following surgical or traumatic loss of a portion or all of one or both maxillary bones and contiguous alveolar structures (e.g., gingival tissue, teeth).

Frequent revisions of surgical obturators are necessary during the ensuing healing phase (approximately six months). Some dentists prefer to replace many or all teeth removed by the surgical procedure in the surgical obturator, while others do not replace any teeth. Further surgical revisions may require fabrication of another surgical obturator (e.g., an initially planned small defect may be revised and greatly enlarged after the final pathology report indicates margins are not free of tumor).

D5932   obturator prosthesis, definitive

Synonymous terminology: obturator

A prosthesis, which artificially replaces part or all of the maxilla and associated teeth, lost due to surgery, trauma or congenital defects.

A definitive obturator is made when it is deemed that further tissue changes or recurrence of tumor are unlikely and a more permanent prosthetic rehabilitation can be achieved; it is intended for long-term use.

● new procedure code   ▲ revision to a nomenclature or descriptor

D5933 obturator prosthesis, modification

Synonymous terminology: adjustment, denture adjustment, temporary or office reline.

Revision or alteration of an existing obturator (surgical, interim, or definitive); possible modifications include relief of the denture base due to tissue compression, augmentation of the seal or peripheral areas to effect adequate sealing or separation between the nasal and oral cavities.

D5934 mandibular resection prosthesis with guide flange

Synonymous terminology: resection device, resection appliance.

A prosthesis which guides the remaining portion of the mandible, left after a partial resection, into a more normal relationship with the maxilla. This allows for some tooth-to-tooth or an improved tooth contact. It may also artificially replace missing teeth and thereby increase masticatory efficiency.

D5935 mandibular resection prosthesis without guide flange

A prosthesis which helps guide the partially resected mandible to a more normal relation with the maxilla allowing for increased tooth contact. It does not have a flange or ramp, however, to assist in directional closure. It may replace missing teeth and thereby increase masticatory efficiency.

Dentists who treat mandibulectomy patients may prefer to replace some, all or none of the teeth in the defect area. Frequently, the defect's margins preclude even partial replacement. Use of a guide (a mandibular resection prosthesis with a guide flange) may not be possible due to anatomical limitations or poor patient tolerance. Ramps, extended occlusal arrangements and irregular occlusal positioning relative to the denture foundation frequently preclude stability of the prostheses, and thus some prostheses are poorly tolerated under such adverse circumstances.

D5936 obturator prosthesis, interim
Synonymous terminology: immediate postoperative obturator.

A prosthesis which is made following completion of the initial healing after a surgical resection of a portion or all of one or both the maxillae; frequently many or all teeth in the defect area are replaced by this prosthesis. This prosthesis replaces the surgical obturator, which is usually inserted at, or immediately following the resection.

Generally, an interim obturator is made to facilitate closure of the resultant defect after initial healing has been completed. Unlike the surgical obturator, which usually is made prior to surgery and frequently revised in the operating room during surgery, the interim obturator is made when the defect margins are clearly defined and further surgical revisions are not planned. It is a provisional prosthesis, which may replace some or all lost teeth, and other lost bone and soft tissue structures. Also, it frequently must be revised (termed an obturator prosthesis modification) during subsequent dental procedures (e.g., restorations, gingival surgery) as well as to compensate for further tissue shrinkage before a definitive obturator prosthesis is made.

D5937 trismus appliance (not for TMD treatment)
Synonymous terminology: occlusal device for mandibular trismus, dynamic bite opener.

A prosthesis, which assists the patient in increasing their oral aperture width in order to eat as well as maintain oral hygiene.

Several versions and designs are possible, all intending to ease the severe lack of oral opening experienced by many patients immediately following extensive intraoral surgical procedures.

D5951 feeding aid
Synonymous terminology: feeding prosthesis.

A prosthesis, which maintains the right and left maxillary segments of an infant cleft palate patient in their proper orientation until surgery is performed to repair the cleft. It closes the oral-nasal cavity defect, thus enhancing sucking and swallowing.

Used on an interim basis, this prosthesis achieves separation of the oral and nasal cavities in infants born with wide clefts necessitating delayed closure. It is eliminated if surgical closure can be effected

● new procedure code   ▲ revision to a nomenclature or descriptor

or, alternatively, with eruption of the deciduous dentition a pediatric speech aid may be made to facilitate closure of the defect.

D5952   speech aid prosthesis, pediatric

Synonymous terminology: nasopharyngeal obturator, speech appliance, obturator, cleft palate appliance, prosthetic speech aid, speech bulb.

A temporary or interim prosthesis used to close a defect in the hard and/or soft palate. It may replace tissue lost due to developmental or surgical alterations. It is necessary for the production of intelligible speech.

Normal lateral growth of the palatal bones necessitates occasional replacement of this prosthesis. Intermittent revisions of the obturator section can assist in maintenance of palatalpharyngeal closure (termed a speech aid prosthesis modification). Frequently, such prostheses are not fabricated before the deciduous dentition is fully erupted since clasp retention is often essential.

D5953   speech aid prosthesis, adult

Synonymous terminology: prosthetic speech appliance, speech aid, speech bulb.

A definitive prosthesis, which can improve speech in adult cleft palate patients either by obturating (sealing off) a palatal cleft or fistula, or occasionally by assisting an incompetent soft palate. Both mechanisms are necessary to achieve velopharyngeal competency.

Generally, this prosthesis is fabricated when no further growth is anticipated and the objective is to achieve long-term use. Hence, more precise materials and techniques are utilized. Occasionally such procedures are accomplished in conjunction with precision attachments in crown work undertaken on some or all maxillary teeth to achieve improved aesthetics.

D5954   palatal augmentation prosthesis

Synonymous terminology: superimposed prosthesis, maxillary glossectomy prosthesis, maxillary speech prosthesis, palatal drop prosthesis.

A removable prosthesis which alters the hard and/or soft palate's topographical form adjacent to the tongue.

D5955 **palatal lift prosthesis, definitive**

A prosthesis which elevates the soft palate superiorly and aids in restoration of soft palate functions which may be lost due to an acquired, congenital or developmental defect.

A definitive palatal lift is usually made for patients whose experience with an interim palatal lift has been successful, especially if surgical alterations are deemed unwarranted.

D5958 **palatal lift prosthesis, interim**

Synonymous terminology: diagnostic palatal lift.

A prosthesis which elevates and assists in restoring soft palate function which may be lost due to clefting, surgery, trauma or unknown paralysis. It is intended for interim use to determine its usefulness in achieving palatalpharyngeal competency or enhance swallowing reflexes.

This prosthesis is intended for interim use as a diagnostic aid to assess the level of possible improvement in speech intelligibility. Some clinicians believe use of a palatal lift on an interim basis may stimulate an otherwise flaccid soft palate to increase functional activity, subsequently lessening its need.

D5959 **palatal lift prosthesis, modification**

Synonymous terminology: revision of lift, adjustment.

Alterations in the adaptation, contour, form or function of an existing palatal lift necessitated due to tissue impingement, lack of function, poor clasp adaptation or the like.

D5960 **speech aid prosthesis, modification**

Synonymous terminology: adjustment, repair, revision.

Any revision of a pediatric or adult speech aid not necessitating its replacement.

Frequently, revisions of the obturating section of any speech aid are required to facilitate enhanced speech intelligibility. Such revisions or repairs do not require complete remaking of the prosthesis, thus extending its longevity.

D5982 surgical stent

Synonymous terminology: periodontal stent, skin graft stent, columellar stent.

Stents are utilized to apply pressure to soft tissues to facilitate healing and prevent cicatrization or collapse.

A surgical stent may be required in surgical and post-surgical revisions to achieve close approximation of tissues. Usually such materials as temporary or interim soft denture liners, gutta percha, or dental modeling impression compound may be used.

D5983 radiation carrier

Synonymous terminology: radiotherapy prosthesis, carrier prosthesis, radiation applicator, radium carrier, intracavity carrier, intracavity applicator.

A device used to administer radiation to confined areas by means of capsules, beads or needles of radiation emitting materials such as radium or cesium. Its function is to hold the radiation source securely in the same location during the entire period of treatment.

Radiation oncologists occasionally request these devices to achieve close approximation and controlled application of radiation to a tumor deemed amiable to eradication.

D5984 radiation shield

Synonymous terminology: radiation stent, tongue protector, lead shield.

An intraoral prosthesis designed to shield adjacent tissues from radiation during orthovoltage treatment of malignant lesions of the head and neck region.

D5985 radiation cone locator

Synonymous terminology: docking device, cone locator.

A prosthesis utilized to direct and reduplicate the path of radiation to an oral tumor during a split course of irradiation.

D5986 fluoride gel carrier

Synonymous terminology: fluoride applicator.

A prosthesis, which covers the teeth in either dental arch and is used to apply topical fluoride in close proximity to tooth enamel and dentin for several minutes daily.

D5987   commissure splint
Synonymous terminology: lip splint.

A device placed between the lips, which assists in achieving increased opening between the lips. Use of such devices enhances opening where surgical, chemical or electrical alterations of the lips has resulted in severe restriction or contractures.

D5988   surgical splint
Synonymous terminology: Gunning splint, modified Gunning splint, labiolingual splint, fenestrated splint, Kingsley splint, cast metal splint.

Splints are designed to utilize existing teeth and/or alveolar processes as points of anchorage to assist in stabilization and immobilization of broken bones during healing. They are used to re-establish, as much as possible, normal occlusal relationships during the process of immobilization. Frequently, existing prostheses (e.g., a patient's complete dentures) can be modified to serve as surgical splints. Frequently, surgical splints have arch bars added to facilitate intermaxillary fixation. Rubber elastics may be used to assist in this process. Circummandibular eyelet hooks can be utilized for enhanced stabilization with wiring to adjacent bone.

D5991   topical medicament carrier
A custom fabricated carrier that covers the teeth and alveolar mucosa, or alveolar mucosa alone, and is used to deliver topical corticosteroids and similar effective medicaments for maximum sustained contact with the alveolar ridge and/or attached gingival tissues for the control and management of immunologically mediated vesiculobullous mucosal, chronic recurrent ulcerative, and other desquamative diseases of the gingiva and oral mucosa.

D5992   adjust maxillofacial prosthetic appliance, by report

D5993   maintenance and cleaning of a maxillofacial prosthesis (extra or intraoral) other than required adjustments, by report
Maintenance and cleaning of a maxillofacial prosthesis.

D5999   unspecified maxillofacial prosthesis, by report
Used for procedure that is not adequately described by a code. Describe procedure.

● new procedure code   ▲ revision to a nomenclature or descriptor

D6000-D6199   VIII. Implant Services

Local anesthesia is usually considered to be part of Implant Services procedures.

Pre-Surgical Services

D6190   radiographic/surgical implant index, by report
An appliance, designed to relate osteotomy or fixture position to existing anatomic structures, to be utilized during radiographic exposure for treatment planning and/or during osteotomy creation for fixture installation.

Surgical Services

Report surgical implant procedure using codes in this section.

D6010   surgical placement of implant body: endosteal implant
Includes second stage surgery and placement of healing cap.

D6012   surgical placement of interim implant body for transitional prosthesis: endosteal implant
Includes removal during later therapy to accommodate the definitive restoration, which may include placement of other implants.

D6040   surgical placement: eposteal implant
An eposteal (subperiosteal) framework of a biocompatible material designed and fabricated to fit on the surface of the bone of the mandible or maxilla with permucosal extensions which provide support and attachment of a prosthesis. This may be a complete arch or unilateral appliance. Eposteal implants rest upon the bone and under the periosteum.

D6050   surgical placement: transosteal implant
A transosteal (transosseous) biocompatible device with threaded posts penetrating both the superior and inferior cortical bone plates of the mandibular symphysis and exiting through the permucosa providing support and attachment for a dental prosthesis. Transosteal implants are placed completely through the bone and into the oral cavity from extraoral or intraoral.

Code on Dental Procedures and Nomenclature

D6100 **implant removal, by report**
This procedure involves the surgical removal of an implant.
Describe procedure.

● **D6101** **debridement of a periimplant defect and surface cleaning of exposed implant surfaces, including flap entry and closure**

● **D6102** **debridement and osseous contouring of a periimplant defect; includes surface cleaning of exposed implant surfaces and flap entry and closure**

● **D6103** **bone graft for repair of periimplant defect – not including flap entry and closure or, when indicated, placement of a barrier membrane or biologic materials to aid in osseous regeneration**

● **D6104** **bone graft at time of implant placement**
Placement of a barrier membrane, or biologic materials to aid in osseous regeneration are reported separately.

Implant Supported Prosthetics

Supporting Structures

D6055 **connecting bar – implant supported or abutment supported**
Utilized to stabilize and anchor a prosthesis.

▲ **D6056** **prefabricated abutment – includes modification and placement**
Modification of a prefabricated abutment may be necessary.

▲ **D6057** **custom fabricated abutment – includes placement**
Created by a laboratory process, specific for an individual application.

● **D6051** **interim abutment**
Includes placement and removal. A healing cap is not an interim abutment.

Implant/Abutment Supported Removable Dentures

D6053 **implant/abutment supported removable denture for completely edentulous arch**

D6054 **implant/abutment supported removable denture for partially edentulous arch**

Implant/Abutment Supported Fixed Dentures (Hybrid Prosthesis)

D6078 implant/abutment supported fixed denture for completely edentulous arch

A prosthesis that is retained, supported and stabilized by implants or abutments placed on implants but does not have specific relationships between implant positions and replacement teeth; may be screw retained or cemented; commonly referred to as a "hybrid prosthesis."

D6079 implant/abutment supported fixed denture for partially edentulous arch

A prosthesis that is retained, supported and stabilized by implants or abutments placed on implants but does not have specific relationship between implant positions and replacement teeth; may be screw retained or cemented; commonly referred to as a "hybrid prosthesis".

Single Crowns, Abutment Supported

D6058 abutment supported porcelain/ceramic crown

A single crown restoration that is retained, supported and stabilized by an abutment on an implant; may be screw retained or cemented.

D6059 abutment supported porcelain fused to metal crown (high noble metal)

A single metal-ceramic crown restoration that is retained, supported and stabilized by an abutment on an implant; may be screw retained or cemented.

D6060 abutment supported porcelain fused to metal crown (predominantly base metal)

A single metal-ceramic crown restoration that is retained, supported and stabilized by an abutment on an implant; may be screw retained or cemented.

D6061 abutment supported porcelain fused to metal crown (noble metal)

A single metal-ceramic crown restoration that is retained, supported and stabilized by an abutment on an implant; may be screw retained or cemented.

D6062   abutment supported cast metal crown (high noble metal)
A single cast metal crown restoration that is retained, supported and stabilized by an abutment on an implant; may be screw retained or cemented.

D6063   abutment supported cast metal crown (predominantly base metal)
A single cast metal crown restoration that is retained, supported and stabilized by an abutment on an implant; may be screw retained or cemented.

D6064   abutment supported cast metal crown (noble metal)
A single cast metal crown restoration that is retained, supported and stabilized by an abutment on an implant; may be screw retained or cemented.

D6094   abutment supported crown (titanium)
A single crown restoration that is retained, supported and stabilized by an abutment on an implant. May be cast or milled and is screw retained or cemented.

Single Crowns, Implant Supported

D6065   implant supported porcelain/ceramic crown
A single crown restoration that is retained, supported and stabilized by an implant; may be screw retained or cemented.

D6066   implant supported porcelain fused to metal crown (titanium, titanium alloy, high noble metal)
A single metal-ceramic crown restoration that is retained, supported and stabilized by an implant; may be screw retained or cemented.

D6067   implant supported metal crown (titanium, titanium alloy, high noble metal)
A single cast metal or milled crown restoration that is retained, supported and stabilized by an implant; may be screw retained or cemented.

● new procedure code   ▲ revision to a nomenclature or descriptor

Fixed Partial Denture, Abutment Supported

D6068 **abutment supported retainer for porcelain/ceramic FPD**
A ceramic retainer for a fixed partial denture that gains retention, support and stability from an abutment on an implant; may be screw retained or cemented.

D6069 **abutment supported retainer for porcelain fused to metal FPD (high noble metal)**
A metal-ceramic retainer for a fixed partial denture that gains retention, support and stability from an abutment on an implant; may be screw retained or cemented.

D6070 **abutment supported retainer for porcelain fused to metal FPD (predominantly base metal)**
A metal-ceramic retainer for a fixed partial denture that gains retention, support and stability from an abutment on an implant; may be screw retained or cemented.

D6071 **abutment supported retainer for porcelain fused to metal FPD (noble metal)**
A metal-ceramic retainer for a fixed partial denture that gains retention, support and stability from an abutment on an implant; may be screw retained or cemented.

D6072 **abutment supported retainer for cast metal FPD (high noble metal)**
A cast metal retainer for a fixed partial denture that gains retention, support and stability from an abutment on an implant; may be screw retained or cemented.

D6073 **abutment supported retainer for cast metal FPD (predominantly base metal)**
A cast metal retainer for a fixed partial denture that gains retention, support and stability from an abutment on an implant; may be screw retained or cemented.

D6074 **abutment supported retainer for cast metal FPD (noble metal)**
A cast metal retainer for a fixed partial denture that gains retention, support and stability from an abutment on an implant; may be screw retained or cemented.

D6194 abutment supported retainer crown for FPD titanium)
A retainer for a fixed partial denture that gains retention, support and stability from an abutment on an implant. May be cast or milled and is screw retained or cemented.

Fixed Partial Denture, Implant Supported

D6075 implant supported retainer for ceramic FPD
A ceramic retainer for a fixed partial denture that gains retention, support and stability from an implant; may be screw retained or cemented.

D6076 implant supported retainer for porcelain fused to metal FPD (titanium, titanium alloy, or high noble metal)
A metal-ceramic retainer for a fixed partial denture that gains retention, support and stability from an implant; may be screw retained or cemented.

D6077 implant supported retainer for cast metal FPD (titanium, titanium alloy, or high noble metal)
A cast metal retainer for a fixed partial denture that gains retention, support and stability from an implant; may be screw retained or cemented.

Other Implant Services

D6080 implant maintenance procedures, including removal of prosthesis, cleansing of prosthesis and abutments and reinsertion of prosthesis
This procedure includes a prophylaxis to provide active debriding of the implant and examination of all aspects of the implant system, including the occlusion and stability of the superstructure. The patient is also instructed in thorough daily cleansing of the implant.

D6090 repair implant supported prosthesis, by report
This procedure involves the repair or replacement of any part of the implant supported prosthesis.

● new procedure code   ▲ revision to a nomenclature or descriptor

D6095 repair implant abutment, by report
This procedure involves the repair or replacement of any part of the implant abutment.

D6091 replacement of semi-precision or precision attachment (male or female component) of implant/abutment supported prosthesis, per attachment
This procedure applies to the replaceable male or female component of the attachment.

D6092 recement implant/abutment supported crown

D6093 recement implant/abutment supported fixed partial denture

D6199 unspecified implant procedure, by report
Use for procedure that is not adequately described by a code. Describe procedure.

▲ D6200–D6999   IX. Prosthodontics, fixed

Each retainer and each pontic constitutes a unit in a fixed partial denture.

Local anesthesia is usually considered to be part of Fixed Prosthodontic procedures.

The term "fixed partial denture" replaces the words "bridge" and "bridgework" throughout this section.

Fixed partial denture prosthetic procedures include routine temporary prosthetics. When indicated, interim or provisional codes should be reported separately.

Fixed Partial Denture Pontics

D6205   pontic – indirect resin based composite
Not to be used as a temporary or provisional prosthesis.

D6210   pontic – cast high noble metal

D6211   pontic – cast predominantly base metal

D6212   pontic – cast noble metal

D6214   pontic – titanium

D6240   pontic – porcelain fused to high noble metal

D6241   pontic – porcelain fused to predominantly base metal

D6242   pontic – porcelain fused to noble metal

D6245   pontic – porcelain/ceramic

D6250   pontic – resin with high noble metal

D6251   pontic – resin with predominantly base metal

D6252   pontic – resin with noble metal

▲ **D6253   provisional pontic– further treatment or completion of diagnosis necessary prior to final impression**
Not to be used as a temporary pontic for routine prosthetic fixed partial dentures.

Fixed Partial Denture Retainers – Inlays/Onlays

D6545 retainer – cast metal for resin bonded fixed prosthesis

D6548 retainer – porcelain/ceramic for resin bonded fixed prosthesis

D6600 inlay – porcelain/ceramic, two surfaces

D6601 inlay – porcelain/ceramic, three or more surfaces

D6602 inlay – cast high noble metal, two surfaces

D6603 inlay – cast high noble metal, three or more surfaces

D6604 inlay – cast predominantly base metal, two surfaces

D6605 inlay – cast predominantly base metal, three or more surfaces

D6606 inlay – cast noble metal, two surfaces

D6607 inlay – cast noble metal, three or more surfaces

D6624 inlay – titanium

D6608 onlay – porcelain/ceramic, two surfaces

D6609 onlay – porcelain/ceramic, three or more surfaces

D6610 onlay – cast high noble metal, two surfaces

D6611 onlay – cast high noble metal, three or more surfaces

D6612 onlay – cast predominantly base metal, two surfaces

D6613 onlay – cast predominantly base metal, three or more surfaces

D6614 onlay – cast noble metal, two surfaces

D6615 onlay – cast noble metal, three or more surfaces

D6634 onlay – titanium

● new procedure code   ▲ revision to a nomenclature or descriptor

Fixed Partial Denture Retainers – Crowns

D6710 **crown – indirect resin based composite**
Not to be used as a temporary or provisional prosthesis.

D6720 **crown – resin with high noble metal**

D6721 **crown – resin with predominantly base metal**

D6722 **crown – resin with noble metal**

D6740 **crown – porcelain/ceramic**

D6750 **crown – porcelain fused to high noble metal**

D6751 **crown – porcelain fused to predominantly base metal**

D6752 **crown – porcelain fused to noble metal**

D6780 **crown – ¾ cast high noble metal**

D6781 **crown – ¾ cast predominantly base metal**

D6782 **crown – ¾ cast noble metal**

D6783 **crown – ¾ porcelain/ceramic**

D6790 **crown – full cast high noble metal**

D6791 **crown – full cast predominantly base metal**

D6792 **crown – full cast noble metal**

D6794 **crown – titanium**

▲ **D6793** **provisional retainer crown– further treatment or completion of diagnosis necessary prior to final impression**
Not to be used as a temporary retainer crown for routine prosthetic fixed partial dentures.

Other Fixed Partial Denture Services

D6920 connector bar
A device attached to fixed partial denture retainer or coping which serves to stabilize and anchor a removable overdenture prosthesis.

D6930 recement fixed partial denture

D6940 stress breaker
A non-rigid connector.

D6950 precision attachment
A male and female pair constitutes one precision attachment, and is separate from the prosthesis.

▲ **D6975 coping**
To be used as a definitive restoration when coping is an integral part of a fixed prosthesis.

▲ **D6980 fixed partial denture repair necessitated by restorative material failure**

D6985 pediatric partial denture, fixed
This prosthesis is used primarily for aesthetic purposes.

D6999 unspecified fixed prosthodontic procedure, by report
Used for procedure that is not adequately described by a code. Describe procedure.

● new procedure code   ▲ revision to a nomenclature or descriptor

D7000-D7999   X. Oral and Maxillofacial Surgery

Local anesthesia is usually considered to be part of Oral and Maxillofacial Surgical procedures.

For dental benefit reporting purposes a quadrant is defined as four or more contiguous teeth and/or teeth spaces distal to the midline.

Extractions (Includes Local Anesthesia, Suturing, If Needed, and Routine Postoperative Care)

D7111   extraction, coronal remnants – deciduous tooth
Removal of soft tissue-retained coronal remnants.

D7140   extraction, erupted tooth or exposed root (elevation and/or forceps removal)
Includes routine removal of tooth structure, minor smoothing of socket bone, and closure, as necessary.

Surgical Extractions (Includes Local Anesthesia, Suturing, If Needed, and Routine Postoperative Care)

D7210   surgical removal of erupted tooth requiring removal of bone and/or sectioning of tooth, and including elevation of mucoperiosteal flap if indicated
Includes related cutting of gingiva and bone, removal of tooth structure, minor smoothing of socket bone and closure.

D7220   removal of impacted tooth – soft tissue
Occlusal surface of tooth covered by soft tissue; requires mucoperiosteal flap elevation.

D7230   removal of impacted tooth – partially bony
Part of crown covered by bone; requires mucoperiosteal flap elevation and bone removal.

D7240   removal of impacted tooth – completely bony
Most or all of crown covered by bone; requires mucoperiosteal flap elevation and bone removal.

D7241   removal of impacted tooth – completely bony, with unusual surgical complications
Most or all of crown covered by bone; unusually difficult or complicated due to factors such as nerve dissection required, separate closure of maxillary sinus required or aberrant tooth position.

D7250   surgical removal of residual tooth roots (cutting procedure)
Includes cutting of soft tissue and bone, removal of tooth structure, and closure.

D7251   coronectomy – intentional partial tooth removal
Intentional partial tooth removal is performed when a neurovascular complication is likely if the entire impacted tooth is removed.

Other Surgical Procedures

D7260   oroantral fistula closure
Excision of fistulous tract between maxillary sinus and oral cavity and closure by advancement flap.

D7261   primary closure of a sinus perforation
Subsequent to surgical removal of tooth, exposure of sinus requiring repair, or immediate closure of oroantral or oralnasal communication in absence of fistulus tract.

D7270   tooth reimplantation and/or stabilization of accidentally evulsed or displaced tooth
Includes splinting and/or stabilization.

D7272   tooth transplantation (includes reimplantation from one site to another and splinting and/or stabilization)

D7280   surgical access of an unerupted tooth
An incision is made and the tissue is reflected and bone removed as necessary to expose the crown of an impacted tooth not intended to be extracted.

D7282   mobilization of erupted or malpositioned tooth to aid eruption
To move/luxate teeth to eliminate ankylosis; not in conjunction with an extraction.

● new procedure code   ▲ revision to a nomenclature or descriptor

D7283   placement of device to facilitate eruption of impacted tooth
Placement of an orthodontic bracket, band or other device on an unerupted tooth, after its exposure, to aid in its eruption. Report the surgical exposure separately using D7280.

D7285   biopsy of oral tissue – hard (bone, tooth)
For removal of specimen only. This code involves biopsy of osseous lesions and is not used for apicoectomy/periradicular surgery.

D7286   biopsy of oral tissue – soft
For surgical removal of an architecturally intact specimen only. This code is not used at the same time as codes for apicoectomy/periradicular curettage.

D7287   exfoliative cytological sample collection
For collection of non-transepithelial cytology sample via mild scraping of the oral mucosa.

D7288   brush biopsy – transepithelial sample collection
For collection of oral disaggregated transepithelial cells via rotational brushing of the oral mucosa.

D7290   surgical repositioning of teeth
Grafting procedure(s) is/are additional.

D7291   transseptal fiberotomy/supra crestal fiberotomy, by report
The supraosseous connective tissue attachment is surgically severed around the involved teeth. Where there are adjacent teeth, the transseptal fiberotomy of a single tooth will involve a minimum of three teeth. Since the incisions are within the gingival sulcus and tissue and the root surface is not instrumented, this procedure heals by the reunion of connective tissue with the root surface on which viable periodontal tissue is present (reattachment).

D7292   surgical placement: temporary anchorage device [screw retained plate] requiring surgical flap
Insertion of a temporary skeletal anchorage device that is attached to the bone by screws and requires a surgical flap. Includes device removal.

D7293   surgical placement: temporary anchorage device requiring surgical flap
Insertion of a device for temporary skeletal anchorage when a surgical flap is required. Includes device removal.

D7294   surgical placement: temporary anchorage device without surgical flap

Insertion of a device for temporary skeletal anchorage when a surgical flap is not required. Includes device removal.

D7295   harvest of bone for use in autogenous grafting procedure

Reported in addition to those autogenous graft placement procedures that do not include harvesting of bone.

Alveoloplasty - Surgical Preparation of Ridge

D7310   alveoloplasty in conjunction with extractions – four or more teeth or tooth spaces, per quadrant

The alveoloplasty is distinct (separate procedure) from extractions and/or surgical extractions. Usually in preparation for a prosthesis or other treatments such as radiation therapy and transplant surgery.

D7311   alveoloplasty in conjunction with extractions – one to three teeth or tooth spaces, per quadrant

The alveoloplasty is distinct (separate procedure) from extractions and/or surgical extractions. Usually in preparation for a prosthesis or other treatments such as radiation therapy and transplant surgery.

D7320   alveoloplasty not in conjunction with extractions – four or more teeth or tooth spaces, per quadrant

No extractions performed in an edentulous area. See D7310 if teeth are being extracted concurrently with the alveoloplasty. Usually in preparation for a prosthesis or other treatments such as radiation therapy and transplant surgery.

D7321   alveoloplasty not in conjunction with extractions – one to three teeth or tooth spaces, per quadrant

No extractions performed in an edentulous area. See D7311 if teeth are being extracted concurrently with the alveoloplasty. Usually in preparation for a prosthesis or other treatments such as radiation therapy and transplant surgery.

● new procedure code   ▲ revision to a nomenclature or descriptor

Vestibuloplasty

Any of a series of surgical procedures designed to increase relative alveolar ridge height.

D7340 **vestibuloplasty – ridge extension (secondary epithelialization)**

D7350 **vestibuloplasty – ridge extension (including soft tissue grafts, muscle reattachment, revision of soft tissue attachment and management of hypertrophied and hyperplastic tissue)**
Surgical Excision of Soft Tissue Lesions

Includes non-odontogenic cysts.

D7410 **excision of benign lesion up to 1.25 cm**

D7411 **excision of benign lesion greater than 1.25 cm**

D7412 **excision of benign lesion, complicated**
Requires extensive undermining with advancement or rotational flap closure.

D7413 **excision of malignant lesion up to 1.25 cm**

D7414 **excision of malignant lesion greater than 1.25 cm**

D7415 **excision of malignant lesion, complicated**
Requires extensive undermining with advancement or rotational flap closure

D7465 **destruction of lesion(s) by physical or chemical method, by report**
Examples include using cryo, laser or electro surgery.

Surgical Excision of Intra-Osseous Lesions

D7440 **excision of malignant tumor – lesion diameter up to 1.25 cm**

D7441 **excision of malignant tumor – lesion diameter greater than 1.25 cm**

D7450   **removal of benign odontogenic cyst or tumor – lesion diameter up to 1.25 cm**

D7451   **removal of benign odontogenic cyst or tumor – lesion diameter greater than 1.25 cm**

D7460   **removal of benign nonodontogenic cyst or tumor – lesion diameter up to 1.25 cm**

D7461   **removal of benign nonodontogenic cyst or tumor – lesion diameter greater than 1.25 cm**
Excision of Bone Tissue

D7471   **removal of lateral exostosis (maxilla or mandible)**

D7472   **removal of torus palatinus**

D7473   **removal of torus mandibularis**

D7485   **surgical reduction of osseous tuberosity**

D7490   **radical resection of maxilla or mandible**
Partial resection of maxilla or mandible; removal of lesion and defect with margin of normal appearing bone. Reconstruction and bone grafts should be reported separately.

Surgical Incision

D7510   **incision and drainage of abscess – intraoral soft tissue**
Involves incision through mucosa, including periodontal origins.

D7511   **incision and drainage of abscess – intraoral soft tissue – complicated (includes drainage of multiple fascial spaces)**
Incision is made intraorally and dissection is extended into adjacent fascial space(s) to provide adequate drainage of abscess/cellulitis.

D7520   **incision and drainage of abscess – extraoral soft tissue**
Involves incision through skin.

D7521   **incision and drainage of abscess – extraoral soft tissue – complicated (includes drainage of multiple fascial spaces)**
Incision is made extraorally and dissection is extended into adjacent fascial space(s) to provide adequate drainage of abscess/cellulitis.

D7530 **removal of foreign body from mucosa, skin, or subcutaneous alveolar tissue**

D7540 **removal of reaction producing foreign bodies, musculoskeletal system**
May include, but is not limited to, removal of splinters, pieces of wire, etc., from muscle and/or bone.

D7550 **partial ostectomy/sequestrectomy for removal of non-vital bone**
Removal of loose or sloughed-off dead bone caused by infection or reduced blood supply.

D7560 **maxillary sinusotomy for removal of tooth fragment or foreign body**

Treatment of Fractures - Simple

D7610 **maxilla – open reduction (teeth immobilized, if present)**
Teeth may be wired, banded or splinted together to prevent movement. Surgical incision required for interosseous fixation.

D7620 **maxilla – closed reduction (teeth immobilized, if present)**
No incision required to reduce fracture. See D7610 if interosseous fixation is applied.

D7630 **mandible – open reduction (teeth immobilized, if present)**
Teeth may be wired, banded or splinted together to prevent movement. Surgical incision required to reduce fracture.

D7640 **mandible – closed reduction (teeth immobilized, if present)**
No incision required to reduce fracture. See D7630 if interosseous fixation is applied.

D7650 **malar and/or zygomatic arch – open reduction**

D7660 **malar and/or zygomatic arch – closed reduction**

D7670 **alveolus – closed reduction, may include stabilization of teeth**
Teeth may be wired, banded or splinted together to prevent movement.

D7671   **alveolus – open reduction, may include stabilization of teeth**
Teeth may be wired, banded or splinted together to prevent movement.

D7680   **facial bones – complicated reduction with fixation and multiple surgical approaches**
Facial bones include upper and lower jaw, cheek, and bones around eyes, nose, and ears.

Treatment of Fractures – Compound

D7710   **maxilla – open reduction**
Surgical incision required to reduce fracture.

D7720   **maxilla – closed reduction**

D7730   **mandible – open reduction**
Surgical incision required to reduce fracture.

D7740   **mandible – closed reduction**

D7750   **malar and/or zygomatic arch – open reduction**
Surgical incision required to reduce fracture.

D7760   **malar and/or zygomatic arch – closed reduction**

D7770   **alveolus - open reduction stabilization of teeth**
Fractured bone(s) are exposed to mouth or outside the face. Surgical incision required to reduce fracture.

D7771   **alveolus, closed reduction stabilization of teeth**
Fractured bone(s) are exposed to mouth or outside the face.

D7780   **facial bones – complicated reduction with fixation and multiple surgical approaches**
Surgical incision required to reduce fracture. Facial bones include upper and lower jaw, cheek, and bones around eyes, nose, and ears.

● new procedure code   ▲ revision to a nomenclature or descriptor

Reduction of Dislocation and Management of Other Temporomandibular Joint Dysfunctions.

Procedures that are an integral part of a primary procedure should not be reported separately.

D7810 **open reduction of dislocation**
Access to TMJ via surgical opening.

D7820 **closed reduction of dislocation**
Joint manipulated into place; no surgical exposure.

D7830 **manipulation under anesthesia**
Usually done under general anesthesia or intravenous sedation.

D7840 **condylectomy**
Surgical removal of all or portion of the mandibular condyle (separate procedure).

D7850 **surgical discectomy, with/without implant**
Excision of the intra-articular disc of a joint.

D7852 **disc repair**
Repositioning and/or sculpting of disc; repair of perforated posterior attachment.

D7854 **synovectomy**
Excision of a portion or all of the synovial membrane of a joint.

D7856 **myotomy**
Cutting of muscle for therapeutic purposes (separate procedure).

D7858 **joint reconstruction**
Reconstruction of osseous components including or excluding soft tissues of the joint with autogenous, homologous, or alloplastic materials.

D7860 **arthrotomy**
Cutting into joint (separate procedure).

D7865 **arthroplasty**
Reduction of osseous components of the joint to create a pseudoarthrosis or eliminate an irregular remodeling pattern (osteophytes).

D7870 arthrocentesis
Withdrawal of fluid from a joint space by aspiration.

D7871 non-arthroscopic lysis and lavage
Inflow and outflow catheters are placed into the joint space. The joint is lavaged and manipulated as indicated in an effort to release minor adhesions and synovial vacuum phenomenon as well as to remove inflammation products from the joint space.

D7872 arthroscopy – diagnosis, with or without biopsy

D7873 arthroscopy – surgical: lavage and lysis of adhesions
Removal of adhesions using the arthroscope and lavage of the joint cavities.

D7874 arthroscopy – surgical: disc repositioning and stabilization
Repositioning and stabilization of disc using arthroscopic techniques.

D7875 arthroscopy – surgical: synovectomy
Removal of inflamed and hyperplastic synovium (partial/complete) via an arthroscopic technique.

D7876 arthroscopy – surgical: discectomy
Removal of disc and remodeled posterior attachment via the arthroscope.

D7877 arthroscopy – surgical: debridement
Removal of pathologic hard and/or soft tissue using the arthroscope.

D7880 occlusal orthotic device, by report
Presently includes splints provided for treatment of temporomandibular joint dysfunction.

D7899 unspecified TMD therapy, by report
Used for procedure that is not adequately described by a code. Describe procedure.

Repair of Traumatic Wounds

Excludes closure of surgical incisions.

D7910 **suture of recent small wounds up to 5 cm**
Complicated Suturing (Reconstruction Requiring Delicate Handling of Tissues and Wide Undermining for Meticulous Closure)

Excludes closure of surgical incisions.

D7911 **complicated suture – up to 5 cm**

D7912 **complicated suture – greater than 5 cm**

Other Repair Procedures

D7920 **skin graft (identify defect covered, location and type of graft)**

• **D7921** **collection and application of autologous blood concentrate product**

D7940 **osteoplasty – for orthognathic deformities**
Reconstruction of jaws for correction of congenital, developmental or acquired traumatic or surgical deformity.

D7941 **osteotomy – mandibular rami**

D7943 **osteotomy – mandibular rami with bone graft; includes obtaining the graft**

D7944 **osteotomy – segmented or subapical**
Report by range of tooth numbers within segment.

D7945 **osteotomy – body of mandible**
Surgical section of lower jaw. This includes the surgical exposure, bone cut, fixation, routine wound closure and normal post-operative follow-up care.

D7946 **LeFort I (maxilla - total)**
Surgical section of the upper jaw. This includes the surgical exposure, bone cuts, downfracture, repositioning, fixation, routine wound closure and normal post-operative follow-up care.

D7947   LeFort I (maxilla – segmented)
When reporting a surgically assisted palatal expansion without downfracture, this code would entail a reduced service and should be "by report."

D7948   LeFort II or LeFort III (osteoplasty of facial bones for midface hypoplasia or retrusion)–without bone graft
Surgical section of upper jaw. This includes the surgical exposure, bone cuts, downfracture, segmentation of maxilla, repositioning, fixation, routine wound closure and normal post-operative follow-up care.

D7949   LeFort II or LeFort III – with bone graft
Includes obtaining autografts.

D7950   osseous, osteoperiosteal, or cartilage graft of the mandible or maxilla - autogenous or nonautogenous, by report
This code may be used for ridge augmentation or reconstruction to increase height, width and/or volume of residual alveolar ridge. It includes obtaining autograft and/or allograft material. Placement of a barrier membrane, if used, should be reported separately.

▲ **D7951   sinus augmentation with bone or bone substitutes via a lateral open approach**
The augmentation of the sinus cavity to increase alveolar height for reconstruction of edentulous portions of the maxilla. This procedure is performed via a lateral open approach. This includes obtaining the bone or bone substitutes. Placement of a barrier membrane if used should be reported separately.

● **D7952   sinus augmentation via a vertical approach**
The augmentation of the sinus to increase alveolar height by vertical access through the ridge crest by raising the floor of the sinus and grafting as necessary. This includes obtaining the bone or bone substitutes.

D7953   bone replacement graft for ridge preservation – per site
Osseous autograft, allograft or non-osseous graft is placed in an extraction or implant removal site at the time of the extraction or removal to preserve ridge integrity (e.g., clinically indicated in preparation for implant reconstruction or where alveolar contour is critical to planned prosthetic reconstruction). Membrane, if used should be reported separately.

D7955 repair of maxillofacial soft and/or hard tissue defect
Reconstruction of surgical, traumatic, or congenital defects of the facial bones, including the mandible, may utilize autograft, allograft, or alloplastic materials in conjunction with soft tissue procedures to repair and restore the facial bones to form and function. This does not include obtaining the graft and these procedures may require multiple surgical approaches. This procedure does not include edentulous maxilla and mandibular reconstruction for prosthetic considerations. See code D7950.

D7960 frenulectomy – also known as frenectomy or frenotomy – separate procedure not incidental to another
Surgical removal or release of mucosal and muscle elements of a buccal, labial or lingual frenum that is associated with a pathological condition, or interferes with proper oral development or treatment.

D7963 frenuloplasty
Excision of frenum with accompanying excision or repositioning of aberrant muscle and z-plasty or other local flap closure.

D7970 excision of hyperplastic tissue - per arch

D7971 excision of pericoronal gingiva
Surgical removal of inflammatory or hypertrophied tissues surrounding partially erupted/impacted teeth.

D7972 surgical reduction of fibrous tuberosity

D7980 sialolithotomy
Surgical procedure by which a stone within a salivary gland or its duct is removed, either intraorally or extraorally.

D7981 excision of salivary gland, by report

D7982 sialodochoplasty
Surgical procedure for the repair of a defect and/or restoration of a portion of a salivary gland duct.

D7983 closure of salivary fistula
Surgical closure of an opening between a salivary duct and/or gland and the cutaneous surface, or an opening into the oral cavity through other than the normal anatomic pathway.

D7990 emergency tracheotomy
Surgical formation of a tracheal opening usually below the cricoid cartilage to allow for respiratory exchange.

D7991 coronoidectomy
Surgical removal of the coronoid process of the mandible.

D7995 synthetic graft – mandible or facial bones, by report
Includes allogenic material.

D7996 implant-mandible for augmentation purposes (excluding alveolar ridge), by report

D7997 appliance removal (not by dentist who placed appliance), includes removal of archbar

D7998 intraoral placement of a fixation device not in conjunction with a fracture
The placement of intermaxillary fixation appliance for documented medically accepted treatments not in association with fractures.

D7999 unspecified oral surgery procedure, by report
Used for procedure that is not adequately described by a code. Describe procedure.

D8000-D8999   XI. Orthodontics

Dentition

Primary Dentition: Teeth developed and erupted first in order of time.

Transitional Dentition: The final phase of the transition from primary to adult teeth, in which the deciduous molars and canines are in the process of shedding and the permanent successors are emerging.

Adolescent Dentition: The dentition that is present after the normal loss of primary teeth and prior to cessation of growth that would affect orthodontic treatment.

Adult Dentition: The dentition that is present after the cessation of growth that would affect orthodontic treatment.

All of the following orthodontic treatment codes may be used more than once for the treatment of a particular patient depending on the particular circumstance. A patient may require more than one interceptive procedure or more than one limited procedure depending on their particular problem.

Limited Orthodontic Treatment

Orthodontic treatment with a limited objective, not involving the entire dentition. It may be directed at the only existing problem, or at only one aspect of a larger problem in which a decision is made to defer or forego more comprehensive therapy.

Examples of this type of treatment would be treatment in one arch only to correct crowding, partial treatment to open spaces or upright a tooth for a bridge or implant and partial treatment for closure of a space(s).

D8010   limited orthodontic treatment of the primary dentition

D8020   limited orthodontic treatment of the transitional dentition

D8030   limited orthodontic treatment of the adolescent dentition

D8040   limited orthodontic treatment of the adult dentition

Interceptive Orthodontic Treatment

Treatment using codes for interceptive orthodontic treatment are for procedures to lessen the severity or future effects of a malformation and to eliminate its cause.

An extension of preventive orthodontics that may include localized tooth movement. Such treatment may occur in the primary or transitional dentition and may include such procedures as the redirection of ectopically erupting teeth, correction of isolated dental crossbite or recovery of recent minor space loss where overall space is adequate.

The key to successful interception is intervention in the incipient stages of a developing problem to lessen the severity of the malformation and eliminate its cause. Complicating factors such as skeletal disharmonies, overall space deficiency, or other conditions may require future comprehensive therapy.

Early phases of comprehensive therapy may utilize some procedures that might also be used interceptively, but such procedures are not considered interceptive in those applications.

D8050 **interceptive orthodontic treatment of the primary dentition**

D8060 **interceptive orthodontic treatment of the transitional dentition**

Comprehensive Orthodontic Treatment

These codes should be used when there are multiple phases of treatment provided at different stages of dentofacial development.

For example, the use of an activator is generally stage one of a two-stage treatment. In this situation, placement of fixed appliances will generally be stage two of a two-stage treatment. Both phases should be listed as comprehensive treatment modified by the appropriate stage of dental development.

This is used to report the coordinated diagnosis and treatment leading to the improvement of a patient's craniofacial dysfunction and/or dentofacial deformity including anatomical, functional and aesthetic relationships. Treatment usually, but not necessarily, utilizes fixed orthodontic appliances. Adjunctive procedures, such as extractions, maxillofacial surgery, nasopharyngeal surgery, myofunctional or speech therapy and restorative or periodontal care, may be coordinated disciplines. Optimal care requires long-term consideration of patient's needs and periodic re-evaluation. Treatment may incorporate several phases with specific objectives at various stages of dentofacial development.

D8070 comprehensive orthodontic treatment of the transitional dentition

D8080 comprehensive orthodontic treatment of the adolescent dentition

D8090 comprehensive orthodontic treatment of the adult dentition

Minor Treatment to Control Harmful Habits

D8210 removable appliance therapy
Removable indicates patient can remove; includes appliances for thumb sucking and tongue thrusting.

D8220 fixed appliance therapy
Fixed indicates patient cannot remove appliance; includes appliances for thumb sucking and tongue thrusting.

Other Orthodontic Services

D8660 pre-orthodontic treatment visit

D8670 periodic orthodontic treatment visit (as part of contract)

D8680 orthodontic retention (removal of appliances, construction and placement of retainer(s))

D8690 orthodontic treatment (alternative billing to a contract fee)
Services provided by dentist other than original treating dentist. A method of payment between the provider and responsible party for services that reflect an open-ended fee arrangement.

D8691 repair of orthodontic appliance
Does not include bracket and standard fixed orthodontic appliances. It does include functional appliances and palatal expanders.

D8692 replacement of lost or broken retainer

D8693 **rebonding or recementing; and/or repair, as required, of fixed retainers**

D8999 **unspecified orthodontic procedure, by report**
Used for procedure that is not adequately described by a code.
Describe procedure.

D9000-D9999 XII. Adjunctive General Services

Unclassified Treatment

D9110 palliative (emergency) treatment of dental pain - minor procedure
This is typically reported on a "per visit" basis for emergency treatment of dental pain.

D9120 fixed partial denture sectioning
Separation of one or more connections between abutments and/or pontics when some portion of a fixed prosthesis is to remain intact and serviceable following sectioning and extraction or other treatment. Includes all recontouring and polishing of retained portions.

Anesthesia

D9210 local anesthesia not in conjunction with operative or surgical procedures

D9211 regional block anesthesia

D9212 trigeminal division block anesthesia

D9215 local anesthesia in conjunction with operative or surgical procedures

D9220 deep sedation/general anesthesia – first 30 minutes
Anesthesia time begins when the doctor administering the anesthetic agent initiates the appropriate anesthesia and non-invasive monitoring protocol and remains in continuous attendance of the patient. Anesthesia services are considered completed when the patient may be safely left under the observation of trained personnel and the doctor may safely leave the room to attend to other patients or duties.

The level of anesthesia is determined by the anesthesia provider's documentation of the anesthetic's effects upon the central nervous system and not dependent upon the route of administration.

D9221 deep sedation/general anesthesia – each additional 15 minutes
Anesthesia time begins when the doctor administering the anesthetic agent initiates the appropriate anesthesia and non-invasive monitoring protocol and remains in continuous attendance of the patient. Anesthesia services are considered completed when the patient may be safely left under the observation of trained personnel and the doctor may safely leave the room to attend to other patients or duties.

The level of anesthesia is determined by the anesthesia provider's documentation of the anesthetic's effects upon the central nervous system and not dependent upon the route of administration.

D9230 inhalation of nitrous oxide/analgesia, anxiolysis

D9241 intravenous conscious sedation/analgesia – first 30 minutes
Anesthesia time begins when the doctor administering the anesthetic agent initiates the appropriate anesthesia and non-invasive monitoring protocol and remains in continuous attendance of the patient. Anesthesia services are considered completed when the patient may be safely left under the observation of trained personnel and the doctor may safely leave the room to attend to other patients or duties.

The level of anesthesia is determined by the anesthesia provider's documentation of the anesthetic's effects upon the central nervous system and not dependent upon the route of administration.

D9242 intravenous conscious sedation/analgesia – each additional 15 minutes
Anesthesia time begins when the doctor administering the anesthetic agent initiates the appropriate anesthesia and non-invasive monitoring protocol and remains in continuous attendance of the patient. Anesthesia services are considered completed when the patient may be safely left under the observation of trained personnel and the doctor may safely leave the room to attend to other patients or duties.

The level of anesthesia is determined by the anesthesia provider's documentation of the anesthetic's effects upon the central nervous system and not dependent upon the route of administration.

● new procedure code   ▲ revision to a nomenclature or descriptor

D9248 **non-intravenous conscious sedation**
A medically controlled state of depressed consciousness while maintaining the patient's airway, protective reflexes and the ability to respond to stimulation or verbal commands. It includes non-intravenous administration of sedative and/or analgesic agent(s) and appropriate monitoring.

The level of anesthesia is determined by the anesthesia provider's documentation of the anesthetic's effects upon the central nervous system and not dependent upon the route of administration.

Professional Consultation

D9310 **consultation – diagnostic service provided by dentist or physician other than requesting dentist or physician**
A patient encounter with a practitioner whose opinion or advice regarding evaluation and/or management of a specific problem; may be requested by another practitioner or appropriate source. The consultation includes an oral evaluation. The consulted practitioner may initiate diagnostic and/or therapeutic services.

Professional Visits

D9410 **house/extended care facility call**
Includes visits to nursing homes, long-term care facilities, hospice sites, institutions, etc. Report in addition to reporting appropriate code numbers for actual services performed.

D9420 **hospital or ambulatory surgical center call**
Care provided outside the dentist's office to a patient who is in a hospital or ambulatory surgical center. Services delivered to the patient on the date of service are documented separately using the applicable procedure codes.

D9430 **office visit for observation (during regularly scheduled hours) – no other services performed**

D9440 **office visit – after regularly scheduled hours**

D9450 **case presentation, detailed and extensive treatment planning**
Established patient. Not performed on same day as evaluation.

Drugs

D9610   therapeutic parenteral drug, single administration
Includes single administration of antibiotics, steroids, anti-inflammatory drugs, or other therapeutic medications. This code should not be used to report administration of sedative, anesthetic or reversal agents.

D9612   therapeutic parenteral drugs, two or more administrations, different medications
Includes multiple administrations of antibiotics, steroids, anti-inflammatory drugs or other therapeutic medications. This code should not be used to report administration of sedatives, anesthetic or reversal agents.

This code should be reported when two or more different medications are necessary and should not be reported in addition to code D9610 on the same date.

D9630   other drugs and/or medicaments, by report
Includes, but is not limited to oral antibiotics, oral analgesics, and topical fluoride dispensed in the office for home use; does not include writing prescriptions.

Miscellaneous Services

D9910   application of desensitizing medicament
Includes in-office treatment for root sensitivity. Typically reported on a "per visit" basis for application of topical fluoride. This code is not to be used for bases, liners or adhesives used under restorations.

D9911   application of desensitizing resin for cervical and/or root surface, per tooth
Typically reported on a "per tooth" basis for application of adhesive resins. This code is not to be used for bases, liners, or adhesives used under restorations.

D9920   behavior management, by report
May be reported in addition to treatment provided. Should be reported in 15-minute increments.

● new procedure code   ▲ revision to a nomenclature or descriptor

D9930 treatment of complications (post-surgical) – unusual circumstances, by report
For example, treatment of a dry socket following extraction or removal of bony sequestrum.

D9940 occlusal guard, by report
Removable dental appliances, which are designed to minimize the effects of bruxism (grinding) and other occlusal factors.

D9941 fabrication of athletic mouthguard

D9942 repair and/or reline of occlusal guard

D9950 occlusion analysis - mounted case
Includes, but is not limited to, facebow, interocclusal records tracings, and diagnostic wax-up; for diagnostic casts, see D0470.

D9951 occlusal adjustment – limited
May also be known as equilibration; reshaping the occlusal surfaces of teeth to create harmonious contact relationships between the maxillary and mandibular teeth. Presently includes discing/odontoplasty/enamoplasty. Typically reported on a "per visit" basis. This should not be reported when the procedure only involves bite adjustment in the routine post-delivery care for a direct/indirect restoration or fixed/removable prosthodontics.

D9952 occlusal adjustment – complete
Occlusal adjustment may require several appointments of varying length, and sedation may be necessary to attain adequate relaxation of the musculature. Study casts mounted on an articulating instrument may be utilized for analysis of occlusal disharmony. It is designed to achieve functional relationships and masticatory efficiency in conjunction with restorative treatment, orthodontics, orthognathic surgery, or jaw trauma when indicated. Occlusal adjustment enhances the healing potential of tissues affected by the lesions of occlusal trauma.

D9970 enamel microabrasion
The removal of discolored surface enamel defects resulting from altered mineralization or decalcification of the superficial enamel layer. Submit per treatment visit.

D9971 **odontoplasty 1-2 teeth; includes removal of enamel projections**

▲ **D9972** **external bleaching – per arch – performed in office**

D9973 **external bleaching – per tooth**

D9974 **internal bleaching – per tooth**

● **D9975** **external bleaching for home application, per arch; includes materials and fabrication of custom trays**

D9999 **unspecified adjunctive procedure, by report**
Used for procedure that is not adequately described by a code. Describe procedure.

● new procedure code   ▲ revision to a nomenclature or descriptor

2 Changes to the CDT Code

Changes to the CDT Code

All changes are illustrated in this section, with text additions underlined in blue ink and deleted text ~~stricken through in red ink.~~ There are:

- 35 new codes

- 37 revised codes

- 12 deleted codes

- 7 changes to subcategories

One change has also been made to the Classification of Materials, which is now at the beginning of the CDT Code –

Porcelain/ceramic

Refers to ~~those~~ pressed, fired, polished or milled materials containing predominantly ~~non-metal, non-resin~~ inorganic refractory compounds ~~processed at high temperatures (600C/1112F and above) and pressed, polished or milled~~ – including porcelains, glasses, ceramics and glass-ceramics

As noted in the preface, the CDT Code is divided into twelve Categories of Service and each category begins at the top of a right-hand page in this section of the manual.

D0100-D0999   I. Diagnostic

This Category of Service has undergone two sets of changes.

The first set of changes is addition of one new subcategory with two new procedure codes, as illustrated below –

One (1) subcategory of service

Pre-diagnostic Services

Two (2) procedure codes

D0190   **screening of a patient**
A screening, including state or federally mandated screenings, to determine an individual's need to be seen by a dentist for diagnosis.

D0191   **assessment of a patient**
A limited clinical inspection that is performed to identify possible signs of oral or systemic disease, malformation, or injury, and the potential need for referral for diagnosis and treatment.

The second set of changes are extensive (37) and are all within the "...Diagnostic Imaging..." subcategory, These changes illustrated in their entirety below. Additions are in blue underline, deletions in ~~red strike-though~~, and unchanged text in black.

~~Radiographs/~~Diagnostic Imaging ~~(Including Interpretation)~~

Should be taken only for clinical reasons as determined by the patient's dentist. Should be of diagnostic quality and properly identified and dated. Is a part of the patient's clinical record and the original images should be retained by the dentist. Originals should not be used to fulfill requests made by patients or third-parties for copies of records.

Image Capture with Interpretation

D0210   **intraoral – complete series** of radiographic images ~~(including bitewings)~~
A radiographic survey of the whole mouth, usually consisting of 14-22 periapical and posterior bitewing images intended to display the crowns and roots of all teeth, periapical areas and alveolar bone.

D0220 intraoral – periapical first radiographic image film

D0230 intraoral – periapical each additional radiographic image film

D0240 intraoral – occlusal radiographic image film

D0250 extraoral – first radiographic image

D0260 extraoral – each additional radiographic image film

D0270 bitewing – single radiographic image film

D0272 bitewings – two radiographic images films

D0273 bitewings – three radiographic images films

D0274 bitewings – four radiographic images films

D0277 vertical bitewings – 7 to 8 radiographic images films
This does not constitute a full mouth intraoral radiographic series.

D0290 posterior-anterior or lateral skull and facial bone survey radiographic image film

D0321 other temporomandibular joint radiographic images films, by report

D0330 panoramic radiographic image film

D0340 cephalometric radiographic image film

D0364 cone beam CT capture and interpretation with with limited field of view – less than one whole jaw

D0365 cone beam CT capture and interpretation with field of view of one full dental arch – mandible

D0366 cone beam CT capture and interpretation with field of view of one full dental arch – maxilla, with or without cranium

D0367 cone beam CT capture and interpretation with field of view of both jaws with or without cranium

D0368 cone beam CT capture and interpretation for TMJ series including two or more exposures

D0369 maxillofacial MRI capture and interpretation

D0370 maxillofacial ultrasound capture and interpretation

D0371 sialoendoscopy capture and interpretation

Image Capture Only

Interpretation and Report Performed by a Practitioner Not Associated With the Capture

D0380 cone beam CT image capture with limited field of view – less than one whole jaw

D0381 cone beam CT image capture with field of view of one full dental arch – mandible

D0382 cone beam CT image capture with field of view of one full dental arch – maxilla, with or without cranium

D0383 cone beam CT image capture with field of view of both jaws, with or without cranium

D0384 cone beam CT image capture for TMJ series including two or more exposures

D0385 maxillofacial MRI image capture

D0386 maxillofacial ultrasound image capture

Interpretation and Report Only

Image Capture Performed by a Practitioner Not Associated With Interpretation and Report

D0391 interpretation of diagnostic image by a practitioner not associated with capture of the image, including report

Deletions
Two (2) procedure codes

~~D0360~~ **~~cone beam ct — craniofacial data capture~~**
~~Includes axial, coronal and sagittal data.~~

~~D0362~~ **~~cone beam — two-dimensional image reconstruction using existing data, includes multiple images~~**

D1000–D1999 II. Preventive

Additions
One (1) procedure code

D1208   topical application of fluoride

Revisions
One (1) procedure code

D1206 topical application of fluoride varnish~~; therapeutic application for moderate to high caries risk patients~~ ~~Application of topical fluoride varnish, delivered in a single visit and involving the entire oral cavity. Not to be used for desensitization.~~

Deletions
Two (2) procedure codes

~~D1203   topical application of fluoride – child~~

~~D1204   topical application of fluoride – adult~~

D2000–D2999 III. Restorative

Additions
Five (5) procedure codes

D2990 resin infiltration of incipient smooth surface lesions
Placement of an infiltrating resin restoration for strengthening, stabilizing and/or limiting the progression of the lesion.

D2929 prefabricated porcelain/ceramic crown – primary tooth

D2981 inlay repair necessitated by restorative material failure

D2982 onlay repair necessitated by restorative material failure

D2983 veneer repair necessitated by restorative material failure

Revisions
Five (5) procedure codes

D2710 crown – resin-based composite (indirect)
~~Unfilled or non-reinforced resin crowns should be reported using D2999.~~

D2799 provisional crown – further treatment or completion of diagnosis necessary prior to final impression
~~Crown utilized as an interim restoration of at least six months duration during restorative treatment to allow adequate time for healing or completion of other procedures. This includes, but is not limited to changing vertical dimension, completing periodontal therapy or cracked-tooth syndrome. This is n~~ Not to be used as a temporary crown for a routine prosthetic restoration.

D2940 protective restoration
Direct placement of a ~~temporary~~ restorative material to protect tooth and/or tissue form. This procedure may be used to relieve pain, promote healing, or prevent further deterioration. Not to be used for endodontic access closure, or as a base or liner under restoration.

D2955 **post removal** ~~(not in conjunction with endodontic therapy)~~
~~For removal of posts (e.g., fractured posts); not to be used in conjunction with endodontic retreatment (D3346, D3347, D3348)~~

D2980 **crown repair~~, by report~~ <u>necessitated by restorative material failure</u>**
~~Includes removal of crown, if necessary. Describe procedure.~~

Deletions

None

D3000-D3999   IV. Endodontics

Additions
None

Revisions
Subcategory of Service

Endodontic Retreatment

~~This procedure may include the removal of a post, pin(s), old root canal filling material, and the procedures necessary to prepare the canals and place the canal filling. This includes complete root canal therapy.~~

One (1) procedure code

D3352   apexification/recalcification/pulpal regeneration – interim medication replacement
For visits in which the intra-canal medication is replaced with new medication ~~and~~. Includes any necessary radiographs.

Deletions
None

D4000-D4999   V. Periodontics

Additions
Three (3) procedure codes

D4212   gingivectomy or gingivoplasty to allow access for restorative procedure, per tooth

D4277   free soft tissue graft procedure (including donor site surgery), first tooth or edentulous tooth position in graft

D4278   free soft tissue graft procedure (including donor site surgery), each additional contiguous tooth or edentulous tooth position in same graft site

Revisions
Seven (7) procedure codes

D4210   **gingivectomy or gingivoplasty – four or more contiguous teeth or tooth bounded spaces per quadrant**
~~Involves the excision of the soft tissue wall of the periodontal pocket by either an external or an internal bevel.~~ It is performed to eliminate suprabony pockets ~~after adequate initial preparation, to allow access for restorative dentistry in the presence of suprabony pockets,~~ or to restore normal architecture when gingival enlargements or asymmetrical or unaesthetic topography is evident with normal bony configuration.

D4211   **gingivectomy or gingivoplasty – four or more contiguous teeth or tooth bounded spaces per quadrant**
~~Involves the excision of the soft tissue wall of the periodontal pocket by either an external or an internal bevel.~~ It is performed to eliminate suprabony pockets ~~after adequate initial preparation, to allow access for restorative dentistry in the presence of suprabony pockets,~~ or to restore normal architecture when gingival enlargements or asymmetrical or unaesthetic topography is evident with normal bony configuration.

D4260 **osseous surgery (including flap entry and closure) – four or more contiguous teeth or tooth bounded spaces per quadrant ...**
This procedure modifies the bony support of the teeth by reshaping the alveolar process to achieve a more physiologic form. This ~~may~~ <u>must</u> include the removal of supporting bone (ostectomy) and/or non-supporting bone (osteoplasty). Other procedures may be required concurrent to D4260 and should be reported using their own unique codes.

D4261 **osseous surgery (including flap entry and closure) – one to three contiguous teeth or tooth bounded spaces per quadrant**
This procedure modifies the bony support of the teeth by reshaping the alveolar process to achieve a more physiologic form. This ~~may~~ <u>must</u> include the removal of supporting bone (ostectomy) and/or non-supporting bone (osteoplasty). Other procedures may be required concurrent to D4261 and should be reported using their own unique codes.

D4266 **guided tissue regeneration – resorbable barrier, per site**
<u>This procedure does not include flap entry and closure, or, when indicated, wound debridement, osseous contouring, bone replacement grafts, and placement of biologic materials to aid in osseous regeneration. This procedure can be used for periodontal and peri-implant defects.</u>

~~A membrane is placed over the root surfaces or defect area following surgical exposure and debridement. The mucoperiosteal flaps are then adapted over the membrane and sutured. The membrane is placed to exclude epithelium and gingival connective tissue from the healing wound. This procedure may require subsequent surgical procedures to correct the gingival contours. Guided tissue regeneration may also be carried out in conjunction with bone replacement grafts or to correct deformities resulting from inadequate faciolingual bone width in an edentulous area. When guided tissue regeneration is used in association with a tooth, each site on a specific tooth should be reported separately. Other separate procedures may be required concurrent to D4266 and should be reported using their own unique codes.~~

D4267 **guided tissue regeneration – non-resorbable barrier, per site (includes membrane removal)**
<u>This procedure does not include flap entry and closure, or, when indicated, wound debridement, osseous contouring, bone replacement</u>

grafts, and placement of biologic materials to aid in osseous regeneration. This procedure can be used for periodontal and peri-implant defects.

~~This procedure is used to regenerate lost or injured periodontal tissue by directing differential tissue responses. A membrane is placed over the root surfaces or defect area following surgical exposure and debridement. The mucoperiosteal flaps are then adapted over the membrane and sutured. This procedure does not include flap entry and closure, wound debridement, osseous contouring, bone replacement grafts, or the placement of biologic materials to aid in osseous tissue regeneration. The membrane is placed to exclude epithelium and gingival connective tissue from the healing wound. This procedure requires subsequent surgical procedures to remove the membrane and/or to correct the gingival contours. Guided tissue regeneration may be used in conjunction with bone replacement grafts or to correct deformities resulting from inadequate faciolingual bone width in an edentulous area. When guided tissue regeneration is used in association with a tooth, each site on a specific tooth should be reported separately with this code. When no tooth is present, each site should be reported separately. Other separate procedures may be reported concurrent to D4267 and should be reported using their own unique codes.~~

D4381   **localized delivery of antimicrobial agents via a controlled release vehicle into diseased crevicular tissue, per tooth**~~, by report~~
FDA approved subgingival delivery devices containing antimicrobial medication(s) are inserted into periodontal pockets to suppress the pathogenic microbiota. These devices slowly release the pharmacological agents so they can remain at the intended site of action in a therapeutic concentration for a sufficient length of time.

Deletions
One (1) procedure code

~~**D4271**~~   ~~**free soft tissue graft procedure (including donor site surgery)**~~
~~Gingival or masticatory mucosa is grafted to create or augment the gingiva at another site, with or without root coverage. This graft may also be used to eliminate the pull of frena and muscle attachments, to extend the vestibular fornix, and to correct localized gingival recession.~~

D5000–D5899   VI. Prosthodontics (removable)

Additions
None

Revisions
None

Deletions
None

D5900-D5999 VII. Maxillofacial Prosthetics

Additions
None

Revisions
None

Deletions
None

D6000–D6199 VIII. Implant Services

Additions

Five (5) procedure code

D6101 **debridement of a periimplant defect and surface cleaning of exposed implant surfaces, including flap entry and closure**

D6102 **debridement and osseous contouring of a periimplant defect; includes surface cleaning of exposed implant surfaces and flap entry and closure**

D6103 **bone graft for repair of periimplant defect – not including flap entry and closure or, when indicated, placement of a barrier membrane or biologic materials to aid in osseous regeneration**

D6104 **bone graft at time of implant placement**
Placement of a barrier membrane, or biologic materials to aid in osseous regeneration are reported separately.

D6051 **interim abutment**
Includes placement and removal. A healing cap is not an interim abutment.

Revisions

Two (2) procedure codes

D6056 **prefabricated abutment – includes modification and placement**
~~A connection to an implant body that is a manufactured component, usually made of machined high noble metal, titanium, titanium alloy or ceramic.~~ Modification of a prefabricated abutment may be necessary~~, and is accomplished by altering its shape using dental burrs/diamonds.~~

D6057 **custom fabricated abutment – includes placement**
~~A connection to an implant body that is a fabricated component, usually by~~ Created by a laboratory process, specific for an individual application. ~~A custom abutment is usually fabricated using a casting process and usually is made of noble of high noble metal. A "UCLA" abutment is an example of this type of abutment.~~

Deletions
None

D6200-D6999 IX. Prosthodontics, fixed

Additions
One (1) category of service descriptor

Fixed partial denture prosthetic procedures include routine temporary prosthetics. When indicated, interim or provisional codes should be reported separately.

Revisions
Four (4) procedure codes

D6253   **provisional pontic – further treatment or completion of diagnosis necessary prior to final impression**
~~Pontic utilized as an interim of at least six months duration during restorative treatment to allow adequate time for healing or completion of other procedures. This is n~~Not to be used as a temporary pontic for routine prosthetic fixed partial dentures

D6793   **provisional retainer crown – further treatment or completion of diagnosis necessary prior to final impression**
~~Retainer crown utilized as an interim of at least six months duration during restorative treatment to allow adequate time for healing or completion of other procedures. This is n~~Not to be used as a temporary retainer crown for routine prosthetic fixed partial dentures.

D6975   **coping~~ – metal~~**
To be used as a definitive restoration when coping is an integral part of a fixed prosthesis.

D6980   **fixed partial denture repair~~, by report~~ necessitated by restorative material failure**

Deletions
Seven (7) procedure codes

~~D6254~~ **interim pontic**
~~Pontic used as an interim restoration for a duration of less than six months when a final impression is not made to allow adequate time for healing or completion of definitive treatment planning. This is not a temporary pontic for routine prosthetic fixed partial denture restoration.~~

~~D6795~~ **interim retainer crown**
~~Retainer crown used as an interim restoration for a duration of less than six months when a final impression is not made to allow adequate time for healing or completion of definitive treatment planning. This is not a temporary retainer crown for routine prosthetic fixed partial denture restoration.~~

~~D6970~~ **post and core in addition to fixed partial denture retainer, indirectly fabricated**
~~Post and core are custom fabricated as a single unit.~~

~~D6972~~ **prefabricated post and core in addition to fixed partial denture retainer**

~~D6973~~ **core buildup for retainer; including any pins**

~~D6976~~ **each additional indirectly fabricated post — same tooth**
~~To be used with D6970.~~

~~D6977~~ **each additional prefabricated post — same tooth**
~~To be used with D6972.~~

D7000-D7999 X. Oral and Maxillofacial Surgery

Additions
Two (2) procedure code

D7921 **collection and application of autologous blood concentrate product**

D7952 **sinus augmentation via a vertical approach**
The augmentation of the sinus to increase alveolar height by vertical access through the ridge crest by raising the floor of the sinus and grafting as necessary. This includes obtaining the bone or bone substitutes.

Revisions
One (1) procedure code

D7951 **sinus augmentation with bone or bone substitutes via a lateral open approach**
The augmentation of the sinus cavity to increase alveolar height for reconstruction of edentulous portions of the maxilla. This procedure is performed via a lateral open approach. This includes obtaining the bone or bone substitutes. Placement of a barrier membrane if used should be reported separately.

Deletions
None

D8000-D8999   XI. Orthodontics

Additions
None

Revisions
None

Deletions
None

D9000–D9999 XII. Adjunctive General Services

Additions
One (1) procedure code

D9975 **external bleaching for home application, per arch; includes materials and fabrication of custom trays**

Revisions
One (1) procedure code

D9972 **external bleaching – per arch –** performed in office

Deletions
None

3 Alphabetical Index to the CDT Code

Alphabetic Index to the CDT Code

Term	Code(s)	Page(s)
A		
Abscess, incision and drainage, all types	D7510, D7511, D7520, D7521	68
Abutments	Also see **Retainers**	
for implants	D6056, D6057, D6051	52, 109
Accession of tissue	D0472 – D0474	10 - 11
Acid etch; part of resin procedure	No separate code	
Adhesives, bonding agents (resin and amalgam bonding agents); part of restorative procedure	No separate code	
Adjunctive General Services (Category of Service)	D9000 – D9999	81 - 86
Adjunctive pre-diagnostic test	D0431	10
Adjust prosthetic appliance	D5992	50
Allograft, soft tissue	D4275, D7955	33, 75
Alveoloplasty	D7310, D7311, D7320, D7321	66
Alveolus, fracture	D7670, D7770	69, 70
Amalgam restorations	D2140 – D2161	15
Amalgam and resin bonding agents (part of restorative procedure)	No separate code	
Analgesia	D9230, D9241, D9242	82
non-intravenous conscious sedation	D9248	83
Anchorage device, temporary		
requiring flap	D7293	65
without flap	D7294	66
screw retained plate requiring flap	D7292	65

Term	Code(s)	Page(s)
Anesthesia		
general	D9220, D9221	81, 82
local	D9210, D9215	81
regional	D9211	81
trigeminal division block	D9212	81
Ankyloglossia	None	
Apexification/recalcification	D3351 – D3353	25-26
Apexogenesis	D3222	24
Apically positioned flap	D4245	31
Apicoectomy/periradicular surgery	D3410 – D3426	26-27
Arthrocentesis	D7870	72
Arthroplasty	D7865	71
Arthroscopy	D7872 – D7877	72
Arthrotomy	D7860	71
Assessment of a patient	D0191	7, 91
Athletic mouthguard	D9941	85
Autologous blood concentrate (collection and application)	D7921	73, 113
B		
Bacteriologic studies	D0415	10
Behavior management	D9920	84
Biologic materials	D4265	32

Term	Code(s)	Page(s)
Biopsy		
brush	D7288	65
hard tissue	D7285	65
soft tissue	D7286	65
Bitewing radiographs	D0270 – D0277	8, 92
Bleaching		
external – per arch	D9972	86, 117
external – per tooth	D9973	86
external bleaching for home application	D9975	86, 117
internal – per tooth	D9974	86
Bone fragment (post-surgical removal)	D9930	85
Bone, harvest of	D7295	66
Bone tissue, excision	D7471 – D7490	68
Bonding agents; adhesives (resin and amalgam bonding agents)	No separate code – part of restorative procedure	
Bridge	See **Fixed Partial Dentures**	
Bruxism appliance	D9940	85

C

Caries susceptibility test	D0425	10
Carrier		
fluoride gel	D5986	49
radiation	D5983	49
topical medicament	D5991	50

Term	Code(s)	Page(s)
Case presentation	D9450	83
Cast post and core	D2952	20
each additional (same tooth)	D2953	20
Casts, diagnostic (study models)	D0470	10
Cephalometric image	D0340	8, 92
Collection and application of autologous blood concentrate	D7921	73, 113
Combined connective tissue and double pedicle graft	D4276	33
Complications, post-surgical	D9930	85
Composite resin	**See Resin-based composite** (direct and indirect)	
Comprehensive orthodontics	D8070 – D8090	79
Condylectomy	D7840	71
Cone Beam – CT		
three-dimensional reconstruction	D0363	8
image capture and interpretation	D0364 – D0368	8-9, 92-93
image capture only	D0380 – D0384	9, 93
interpretation and report only	D0391	9, 93
Connector bar		
dental implant supported	D6055	52
fixed partial denture	D6920	62
Conscious sedation	D9241, D9242, D9248	82-83
Consultation	D9310	83

Alphabetical Index to the CDT Code

Term	Code(s)	Page(s)
Cryosurgery	D7465	67
Culture and sensitivity test	D0415	10
Culture, viral	D0416	10
Curettage		
open flap	D4240, D4241	30
without flap	D4341, D4342	34
Cysts, removal of	D7410 – D7465	67
Cytologic smears	D0480	11
Cytology sample collection	D7287	65

D

Debridement		
endodontic	D3221	23
full mouth	D4355	35
periimplant	D6101 – D6102	52
Dentures (removable)		
adjustments	D5410 – D5422	38
complete	D5110 – D5120	37
immediate, complete	D5130, D5140	37
implant/abutment supported, complete	D6053	52
implant/abutment supported, partial	D6054	52
modification of removable prosthesis following implant surgery	D5875	40
overdenture	D5860, D5861	40

Term	Code(s)	Page(s)
Drugs		
therapeutic parenteral, single administration	D9610	84
therapeutic parental, two or more administrations	D9612	84
other	D9630	84
Dry socket/localized osteitis	D9930	85
E		
Emergency treatment	D0140, D9110	5, 81
Enamel microabrasion	D9970	85
Enameloplasty	D9971	86
Endodontics (Category of Service)	D3000 – D3999	23-27, 99
Endodontic endosseous implant	D3460	27
Equilibration	D9951, D9952	85
Eruption of teeth		
mobilization, surgical	D7282	64
placement of device to aid eruption	D7283	65
Evaluations		
periodic – established patient	D0120	5
limited – problem focused	D0140	5
for patient under 3 years & counseling with primary caregiver	D0145	5
comprehensive – new or established patient	D0150	6
detailed and extensive – problem focused, by report	D0160	6

Term	Code(s)	Page(s)
re-evaluation – limited	D0170	6
comprehensive periodontal – new or established patient	D0180	7
Excision		
benign lesion	D7410 – D7412	67
malignant lesion/tumor	D7413 – D7415, D7440, D7441	67
Exfoliative cytological smear	D0480	11
Exostosis (tuberosity); removal of		
lateral exostosis	D7471	68
osseous tuberosity	D7485	68
surgical reduction of fibrous tuberosity	D7972	75
torus palatinus	D7472	68
torus mandibularis	D7473	68
Extraoral Images (radiographic)	D0250, D0260	8, 92
Extractions	D7111, D7140	63
surgical	D7210 – D7250	63-64

F

Facial Bone Survey	D0290	8, 92
Fiberotomy, transseptal	D7291	65
Fibroma	D7410, D7411	67
Fissurotomy	see **Odontoplasty**	
Fistula		
oroantral	D7260	64

Term	Code(s)	Page(s)
salivary	D7983	75
Fixation device, not in conjunction with fracture	D7998	76
Fixed partial dentures (bridges)		
pontics	D6205 – D6253	59, 111
recementation	D6930	62
repair	D6980	62
retainers		
crowns	D6710 – D6794	61
implant/abutment supported	D6068 – D6077, D6194	55-56
inlay/onlay	D6600 – D6634	60
Maryland Bridge	D6545, D6548	60
pediatric	D6985	62
sectioning	D9120	81
Flaps		
apically positioned	D4245	31
gingival	D4240, D4241	30
Flexible base partial denture	D5225, D5226	37
"Flipper", interim/transitional removable prosthesis (aka "stayplate")	D5820, D5821	39-40
Fluoride		
dispensing for home use	D9630	84
gel carrier	D5986	49
topical	D1208	13, 95

Alphabetical Index to the CDT Code

Term	Code(s)	Page(s)
Gingiva, pericoronal, removal of	D7971	75
Gingival flap	D4240, D4241	30
Gingivectomy/gingivoplasty	D4210, D4212	29-30, 101
Glass ionomers (resin restorations)	D2330 – D2394	16
Gold foil	D2410 – D2430	16
Graft		
bone replacement	D4263, D4264, D6103, D6104 D7953	31-32, 52, 74, 109
combined connective tissue and double pedicle	D4276	33
free soft tissue	D4277 – D4278	33-34, 101
maxillofacial soft/hard tissue	D7955	75
osseous, osteoperiosteal, or cartilage	D7950	85, 74
pedicle soft tissue	D4270	33
sinus augmentation	D7951	74, 113
skin	D7920	73
soft tissue	D4270 – D4273	33
subepithelial connective tissue	D4273	33
synthetic	D7955	75
Guided tissue regeneration	D4266, D4267	32, 102

H

Harvest of bone	D7295	66
Hemisection	D3920	27
Hospital call (hospital or ambulatory surgicenter visit)	D9420	83

Term	Code(s)	Page(s)
House call (nursing home visit)	D9410	83
Hyperplastic tissue removal	D7970	75

I

Term	Code(s)	Page(s)
Images, oral/facial	D0350	8
Immediate complete denture	D5130, D5140	37
Impacted tooth, removal of	D7220 – D7241	63-64
Implant		
chin	D7995	76
endodontic	D3460	27
endosteal/endosseous	D6010	51
eposteal/subperiosteal	D6040	51
interim implant	D6012	51
maintenance	D6080	56
mandible	D7996	76
modification of removable prosthesis	D5875	40
other implant services	D6080 – D6199	56-57
radiographic/surgical implant index	D6190	51
recement	D6092, D6093	57
removal	D6100	52
repair	D6090, D6091, D6095	56-57
transosteal/transosseous	D6050	51
Implant Services (Category of Service)	D6000 – D6199	51-57, 109
Implantation (of tooth)	See **Reimplantation**	

Term	Code(s)	Page(s)
Incision and drainage	D7510, D7511, D7520, D7521	68
Inlay		
fixed partial denture retainers		
metallic	D6602 – D6607, D6624	60
porcelain/ceramic	D6600 – D6601	60
metallic	D2510 – D2530	17
porcelain/ceramic	D2610 – D2630	17
recement inlay	D2910	19
resin-based composite	D2650 – D2652	17
Intentional reimplantation	D3470	27
Interceptive orthodontics	D8050, D8060	78
Interim abutment	D6051	52, 109
Interim complete denture	D5810, D5811	39
Interim partial denture	D5820, D5821	39-40
Internal root repair	D3333	25
Interpretation of diagnostic image (different practitioner)	D0391	9, 93
Intravenous conscious sedation/analgesia		
first 30 minutes	D9241	82
each additional 15 minutes	D9242	82

J

Term	Code(s)	Page(s)
Joint reconstruction	D7858	71

Term	Code(s)	Page(s)
K		
No "K" terms		
L		
Labial veneer	D2960, D2961, D2962	20
Laser	No separate code – part of dental procedure code that appropriately describes the service provided	
Lateral exostosis	D7471	68
LeFort I, osteotomy	D7946, D7947	73-74
II, osteotomy	D7948, D7949	74
III, osteotomy	D7948, D7949	74
Lesions, surgical excision		
intra-osseous lesions	D7440 – D7461	67-68
soft tissue	D7410 – D7415, D7465	67
Limited orthodontic treatment	D8010 – D8040	77
Localized osteitis/dry socket	D9930	85
M		
Maintenance and cleaning of prosthesis	D5993	50
Malar bone, repair of fracture	D7650, D7660, D7750, D7760	69-70
Malocclusion, correction of	D8000 – D8999	77-80
Mandible, fracture of	D7630 – D7640, D7730 – D7740	69-70
Maryland Bridge (resin bonded fixed prosthesis)		
retainer/abutment	D6545, D6548	60

Term	Code(s)	Page(s)
pontic	D6210 – D6252	59
Maxilla, repair of fracture	D7610 – D7620, D7710 – D7720	69-70
Maxillofacial defect	D7955	75
Maxillofacial MRI		
capture and interpretation	D0369	9, 93
image capture (only)	D0385	9, 93
Maxillofacial Prosthodontics (Category of Service)	D5900 - D5999	41-50
adjust prosthetic appliance	D5992	50
maintenance and cleaning of prosthesis	D5993	50
Maxillofacial ultrasound		
capture and interpretation	D0370	9, 93
image capture (only)	D0386	9, 93
Metals, classification of		4
Microabrasion, enamel	D9970	85
Microorganisms, culture and sensitivity	D0415	10
Moulage, facial	D5911, D5912	41
Mouthguard, athletic	D9941	85
Mucosal abnormalities, pre-diagnostic test	D0431	10
Myotomy	D7856	71

N

Neoplasms, removal of	D7410 – D7465	67
Nightguard	D9940	85

Term	Code(s)	Page(s)
Nitrous oxide, analgesia	D9230	82
Non-intravenous conscious sedation	D9248	83
Non-odontogenic cyst	D7460, D7461	68
Nursing home, (house/extended care facility visit)	D9410	83
Nutritional counseling	D1310	13

O

Obturator		
post surgical	D5932	44
refitting	D5933	45
surgical	D5931	44
Occlusal adjustment (equilibration)	D9951, D9952	85
Occlusal image, intraoral	D0240	7, 92
Occlusal guard	D9940	85
reline or repair	D9942	85
Occlusal orthotic device	D7880	72
Occlusion analysis	D9950	85
Odontogenic cyst	D7450, D7451	68
Odontoplasty (enameloplasty)	D9971	86
Office visit	D9430, D9440	83
Onlay		
fixed partial denture retainers, metallic	D6610 – D6615, D6634	60
metallic	D2542 – D2544	17

Term	Code(s)	Page(s)
Osteitis, localized; dry socket	D9930	85
Osteoplasty	D7940	73
Osteotomy	D7941 – D7945	73
Overdenture	D5860, D5861	40
dental implant supported fixed	D6078, D6079	53
dental implant supported removable	D6053, D6054	52
P		
Palliative treatment	D9110	81
Panoramic image	D0330	8, 92
Partial dentures, fixed	See **fixed partial denture**	
Partial dentures, removable		
adjustments	D5421, D5422	38
cast metal framework, resin base	D5213, D5214	37
flexible base	D5225, D5226	37-38
implant/abutment supported	D6054	52
interim	D5820, D5821	39-40
overdenture	D5861	40
reline	D5740, D5741, D5760, D5761	39
repair	D5610 – D5671	38
resin base	D5211, D5212	37
unilateral	D5281	38

Term	Code(s)	Page(s)
Patient		
Screening	D0190	7, 91
Assessment	D0191	7, 91
Perforation defect, internal repair	D3333	25
Periapical images	D0220 - D0230	7, 92
Pericoronal gingival excision	D7971	75
Periodontal evaluation	D0180	7
Periodontal maintenance	D4910	35
Periodontics (Category of Service)	D4000 – D4999	29-35, 101
Periradicular surgery/apicoectomy	D3410 – D3426	26-27
Pharmacologic agents	See **Drugs**	
Photographic images, diagnostic	D0350	8
Pin retention	D2951	19
Pit and fissure sealant	D1351	14
Plasma rich protein	D4265	32
Porcelain/ceramic, definition of		4
Post and core		
indirectly fabricated	D2952	20
each additional (same tooth)	D2953	20
prefabricated	D2954	20
each additional (same tooth)	D2957	20
Post, removal of	D2955	20
Precision attachment	D5862, D6950	40, 62

Term	Code(s)	Page(s)
Replacement of replaceable part	D5867, D6091	40, 57
Prefabricated crown	D2929 – D2933	19, 97
Preventive (Category of Service)	D1000 – D1555	13-14, 95
Preventive resin restoration	D1352	14
Prophylaxis	D1110, D1120	13
Prostheses (maxillofacial prosthetics)	D5900 – D5999	44-50
auricular	D5914	41
cranial	D5924	43
mandibular resection	D5934, D5935	45
ocular	D5916	42
orbital	D5915	42
palatal	D5954 – D5959	47-48
speech aid	D5952, D5953, D5960	47-48
Prosthodontics		
fixed (Category of Service)	D6200 – D6999	59-62
implant-supported	D6053 – D6079, D6094, D6194	52-54, 56
maxillofacial	D5900 – D5999	41-50
removable (Category of Service)	D5000 – D5899	37-40
Protective restoration	D2940	19, 97
Provisional		
single crown	D2799	18
pontic (FPD)	D6253	59, 111
retainer crown (FPD)	D6793	61, 111

Term	Code(s)	Page(s)
Recement		
bridge	D6930	62
crown	D2920	19
fixed retainers	D8693	80
implant fixed partial denture	D6093	57
implant crown	D6092	57
inlay	D2910	19
onlay	D2910	19
post and core	D2915	19
space maintainer	D1550	14
veneer	D2910	19
Reimplantation		
intentional	D3470	27
accidentally evulsed or displaced	D7270	64
Removable partial denture	See **Partial Dentures**	
Repair		
complete removable denture	D5510, D5520	38
crown	D2980	21, 98
fixed partial denture	D6980	62, 111
implant precision or semi-precision attachment	D6091	57
inlay	D2981	21, 97
occlusal guard	D9942	85
onlay	D2982	21, 97

Alphabetical Index to the CDT Code

Term	Code(s)	Page(s)
orthodontic appliance	D8691	79
orthodontic fixed retainer	D8693	80
precision or semi-precision attachment	D5867	40
removable partial dentures	D5610 - D5671	38
veneer	D2983	21, 97
Resin, definition of		4
Resin-based composite, direct		
anterior	D2330 – D2335	16
crown	D2390	16
posterior	D2391 – D2394	16
veneers	D2960	20
Resin-based composite, indirect		
crown	D2710	18, 97
fixed partial denture abutment	D6710	61
inlay/onlay	D2650 – D2664	17
pontic	D6205	59
¾ crown	D2712	18
veneers	D2961	20
Restorations		
amalgam	D2140 – D2161	15
gold foil	D2410 – D2430	16
inlay/onlay	D2510 – D2664,	17
	D6600 – D6634	60

Term	Code(s)	Page(s)
resin-based composite	D2330 – D2394	16
resin infiltration	D2990	19, 97
preventive resin	D1352	14
protective	D2940	19, 97
Restorative (Category of Service)	D2000 – D2999	15-21, 97
Retainers		
fixed partial denture		
resin bonded (aka "Maryland Bridge")	D6545, D6548	60
inlays/onlays	D6600 – D6634	60
crowns	D6710 – D6794	61
implant abutment supported	D6068 – D6074, D6194	55-56
implant supported	D6075 – D6077	56
orthodontic	D8680	79
Retreatment, endodontic	D3346 – D3348	25, 99
Retrograde filling	D3430	27
Revision, periodontal surgery	D4268	32
Ridge augmentation (grafting)	D7950	74
Root		
planing	D4341	34
removal	D7140, D7250	63-64
resection/amputation	D3450	27
Root canal		
therapy	D3310 – D3353	24-26

Term	Code(s)	Page(s)
obstruction	D3331	25
incomplete	D3332	25
Rubber dam, surgical isolation	D3910	27

S

Saliva		
sample collection	D0417	10
analysis of sample	D0418	10
Salivary gland		
excision	D7981	75
fistula closure	D7983	75
Scaling and root planing	D4341, D4342	34
Screening of a patient	D0190	7, 91
Sealant	D1351	14
Section of fixed partial denture	D9120	81
Sedation		
deep	D9220, D9221	81-82
intravenous, conscious	D9241, D9242	82
non-intravenous, conscious	D9248	83
Sedative filling	See **Protective Restoration**	
Sequestrectomy	D7550	69
Sialodochoplasty	D7982	75
Sialoendoscopy capture and interpretation	D0371	9, 93

Term	Code(s)	Page(s)
Sialography	D0310	8
Sialolithotomy	D7980	75
Sinus augmentation		
via lateral open approach	D7951	74, 113
via vertical approach	D7952	74, 113
Sinus perforation, closure	D7261	64
Sinusotomy	D7560	69
Skin graft	D7920	73
Sleep apnea appliance	D5999	50
Space maintainer	D1510 – D1550	14
recement	D1550	14
removal (by dentist who did not place appliance)	D1555	14
Speech aid		
adult	D5953	47
pediatric	D5952	47
Splinting		
commissure	D5987	50
provisional	D4320, D4321	34
surgical	D5988	50
Stainless steel crown	D2930, D2931, D2933, D2934	19
Stayplate (aka "flipper")	D5820, D5821	39-40
Stent	D5982	49

Term	Code(s)	Page(s)
Stress breaker	D6940	62
Supra crestal fiberotomy	D7291	65
Surgical/ambulatory center	D9420	83
Suturing		
simple	D7910	73
complicated	D7911, D7912	73
Synovectomy	D7854	71

T

Temporomandibular joint (TMJ)		
radiographs	D0320, D0321	8, 92
treatment	D7810 – D7899	71-72
Thumb sucking appliance	D8210, D8220	79
Tissue conditioning	D5850, D5851	40
Tissue, excision of hyperplastic	D7970	75
Titanium		
crown, FPD retainer	D6794	61
crown, single unit	D2794	18
implant, abutment supported	D6094	54
implant, abutment supported for FPD	D6194	56
implant supported	D6065	54
implant supported for FPD	D6067	54
inlay, FPD retainer	D6624	60

Term	Code(s)	Page(s)
onlay, FPD retainer	D6634	60
pontic	D6214	59
Tobacco counseling	D1320	13
Tomographic survey	D0322	8
Tongue thrusting appliance	D8210, D8220	79
Tooth, natural		
caries susceptibility test	D0425	10
extraction	D7111, D7140, D7210 – D7250	63-64
impacted, removal of	D7220 – D7241	63-64
intentional reimplantation	D3470	27
pulp vitality test	D0460	10
reimplantation, evulsed/displaced	D7270	64
surgical access	D7280	64
surgical repositioning	D7290	65
transplantation	D7272	64
Topical medicament carrier	D5991	50
Torus (removal of)		
mandibularis	D7473	68
palatinus	D7472	68
Tracheotomy, emergency	D7990	76
Transplantation, tooth	D7272	64
Transseptal fiberotomy	D7291	65

Term	Code(s)	Page(s)
Trismus appliance	D5937	46
Tuberosity		
fibrous	D7972	75
surgical reduction	D7485	68
Tumors, (removal of)	D7440 – D7465	67
U		
Unerupted tooth, surgical access	D7280	64
Unilateral removable partial denture	D5281	38
V		
Veneers	D2960 – D2962	20
Vertical bitewings	D0277	8, 92
Vestibuloplasty	D7340, D7350	67
Viral culture	D0416	10
W		
Wax-up (diagnostic)	D9950	85
Whitening	See **Bleaching**	
Wounds, treatment of	D7910 – D7912	73
X		
X-rays	See **Diagnostic Imaging**	
Y		
No "Y" terms.		

Term	Code(s)	Page(s)
Z		
Zygomatic arch		
simple fracture treatment		
open reduction	D7650	69
closed reduction	D7660	69
compound fracture treatment		
open reduction	D7750	70
closed reduction	D7760	70

4 Guide to the CDT Manual CD-ROM

Guide to the CDT Manual CD-ROM

The CD-ROM included with this book contains the complete text of the American Dental Association's *CDT 2013: Current Dental Terminology* in electronic format. The *CDT* CD-ROM makes it easy for computer users to find the most up-to-date dental codes and definitions. Benefits of the CD-ROM include:

- menu and bookmarks to quickly navigate between sections
- searchable text to locate specific terms and codes
- PDF files to save on your computer so the Code is always at your fingertips

CD-ROM Compatibility with Your Computer

This CD-ROM will run on computers with the Windows XP with Service Pack 3 operating system and newer versions. You will need to reinsert the CD-ROM each time you wish to run the program. The CD-ROM menu will only function on Macs running Parallels or a similar PC emulation product. If you are on a Mac but do not run one of these programs, you can still open files directly from the CD-ROM via the CD-ROM directory (see "Starting the CD-ROM" section below).

The documents on this CD-ROM are provided in Adobe® PDF format. To view them, you will need **Adobe® Acrobat® Reader** version 7.0 or higher. If you do not have this software, you can download it for free at *http://www.adobe.com/ products/reader.html*. You can also install it on your computer (or test to see if you have it) from the CD-ROM menu.

Starting the CD-ROM

Insert the CD-ROM into your computer's CD-ROM drive.

- If you are using **Windows,** the menu may appear automatically after the title screen. If it does not, click on the Windows **Start** menu, select **Run,** and type in D:\cdt2013.exe (where "D" is you CD-ROM drive). The menu page will then appear. Just click on the heading of the document you'd like to view.

- If you are using a **Mac,** double-click on the "CDT 2013" CD icon on your desktop. A window will open and you can double-click on either the "CDT 2013 PDFs" folder to view the book chapter by chapter.

Navigating Documents

Once opened, the PDF files will look like the pages of the CDT manual. You can turn on the Bookmarks feature of an open PDF document by clicking on the **Bookmarks** tab in the upper left corner. Each bookmark is a link to the corresponding section of the document.

To get back to the Menu page, click on the **CDT icon** on the status bar at the bottom of the page, or close the Reader window.

All PDF documents on the CD-ROM are searchable. There are two main ways to **locate a keyword or code** within the text of a document:

- To **Find** the next appearance of a term, hit Ctrl + F, type the search term and hit Enter. Or, choose Edit from the Menu bar, then Find. The Find function only looks for the term in the current document.

- To **Search** for all instances of a term in the document, hit Shift + Ctrl + F and type in the text. This Search function also allows you to search for the term in other documents on the CD-ROM or your computer. For help using Adobe® Acrobat® Reader, open the reader and select **Help** from the top menu bar at the top of your screen. You can also visit the Adobe® website at *www.adobe.com.*

Printing Documents

To print an open PDF document, click on the **Print** icon at the upper left of the page, or choose **File,** then **Print.** The entire chapter will print unless you specify Current Page or give a page range.

Exiting Program

To get out of the program, click on the **Close Window** icon (X at top right of the CD-ROM menu). You will see a message box with a question mark. Select "Exit program" and eject the CD-ROM from the drive.

Questions about CDT Content

For questions about dental procedure coding or claim submission, call the ADA Member Service Center at 800.621.8099. Support is available 8:30 a.m. to 5:00 p.m. CST, Monday through Friday.

Computer/CD Technical Support

For technical support regarding the *CDT 2013 CD-ROM,* call the ADA Technical Support Center toll free at 800.232.2165. Support is available 8:30 a.m. to 5:00 p.m. CST, Monday through Friday.